THE
LIVER DETOX
PLAN

*The Revolutionary Way to
Cleanse and Revive your Body and
Normalise your Weight*

Xandria Williams

Vermilion
LONDON

13 15 17 19 18 16 14

Text copyright © Xandria Williams 1998

The right of Xandria Williams to be identified as the author of this book
has been asserted by her in accordance with the Copyright, Designs and
Patents Act, 1988.

First published in the United Kingdom in 1998 by Vermilion
an imprint of Ebury Press
Random House,
20 Vauxhall Bridge Road,
London SW1V 2SA

Random House Australia (Pty) Limited
20 Alfred Street, Milsons Point, Sydney,
New South Wales 2061, Australia

Random House New Zealand Limited
18 Poland Road, Glenfield,
Auckland 10, New Zealand

Random House South Africa (Pty) Limited
Isle of Houghton, Corner of Boundary Road & Carse O'Gowrie,
Houghton 2198, South Africa

Random House Publishers India Private Limited
301 World Trade Tower, Hotel Intercontinental Grand Complex,
Barakhamba Lane, New Delhi 110 001, India

Random House UK Limited Reg. No. 954009

A CIP catalogue record for this book is available from the British Library

ISBN: 9780091816773

Printed and bound in Great Britain by
Mackays of Chatham Ltd, Chatham, Kent

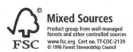

Although every effort has been made to ensure that the contents of
this book are accurate, it must not be treated as a substitute for
qualified medical advice. Always consult a qualified medical
practitioner. Neither the Author nor the Publisher can be held
responsible for any loss or claim arising out of the use, or misuse, of
the suggestions made or the failure to take medical advice.

Xandria Williams, MSC, DIC, ARCS, ND, DBM, MRN
Naturopath, Nutritionist, Herbalist, Homeopath, NLP Practitioner

Xandria Williams began her career as a geochemist, she then turned to bio-chemistry and human nutrition. She is a naturopath, nutritionist, herbalist, homeopath and an NLP practitioner, currently in practice in central London.

She has lectured extensively on nutrition, natural therapies and physical, mental and emotional health care. She lectures in biochemistry and nutrition at the British College of Naturopathy and Osteopathy, and at the Institute of Optimum Nutrition in London.

She has written over 350 articles and 14 books and has appeared frequently on radio and television.

Xandria's unique and highly effective approach to tackling life's problems, physical and emotional, has evolved over more than two decades of writing, research, teaching and helping patients.

Other books available from Xandria Williams:

The Four Temperaments	£8.99
Be happier, have fun and improve relationships by learning about your temperament and that of other people	
Living with allergies	£7.99
How to cope, practically and emotionally	
What's in My Food?	£7.99
Choosing Health Intentionally	£5.99
Choosing Weight Intentionally	£5.99
2 books on the emotional aspects of health and weight control	
Fatigue – The secrets of getting your energy back	£7.99
You're Not Alone	£7.99
Overcoming Candida	£5.99

Ordering:

These books are available from good bookshops or from Xandria Williams.
To obtain copies from Xandria please send a cheque or money order, made payable to XK Williams and include £1.00 per book (max. £3) for postage and handling.

Liver Detox Supplement

The supplement containing all the nutrients discussed in the text is available from Nutri on 01663 747 711

Xandria is currently in practice in central London and can be contacted for consultations.

28 Lower Sloane Street, London SW1W 8BJ
Phone/fax 0171 824 8153, Email xkw@bigfoot.com

Contents

Introduction

I gave considerable thought to the sequence in which the contents of this book would be presented. Initially I favoured a logical and evolving approach, telling you first of all about the liver and what it does when it is healthy, then covering the various things you could be doing and substances you could be consuming that could harm it; this would have led logically on to a discussion of what happens when it goes wrong and the various and *many* consequences to the health of the rest of your body when it does. By then, I hoped, you would have a full understanding as to the way in which many of your current health problems may not be localised problems but may stem from, or be worsened by, an unhealthy liver and a toxic system. At this point, I told myself, you would be so enthused with an understanding for what is happening in your body and the desire to make positive changes that you would willingly enter into the Liver Detox Plan and, moreover, be prepared to stick to it, even when the temptations to digress mount. So in the second half of the book I was then going to give you the full details of the Liver Detox Plan.

But life's not like that. After some careful thought I recognised that many people are not going to sit down and read a book of this sort from cover to cover. You are more likely to dip into it, find something that catches your immediate attention and then want to know what you should do about it, now, so that you can then get on with the rest of your life, feeling healthier and more energetic. For this reason I have rearranged the book into its present format.

You will find, in the next few pages, a broad and sweeping description of what the liver does and the harm you may be suffering if your liver is not as healthy as it should be. Immediately after that comes the programme itself and the information you will need to put it into practice. Only after that, in Section 2, is more detailed information given as to what the liver is, what it does, what harms it and why the suggestions in the programme are being made and the various foods, supplements and remedies being recommended.

Whatever you do, this programme will improve the health of your liver, and that in turn will improve your overall health, well-being and longevity. So let's get started.

SECTION 1

Part I
Overview of the Liver's Role

When, as a biochemist, I first became interested in naturopathy and started talking to naturopathic practitioners it struck me that they had an obsession with finding out about people's bowels and their stools that was bordering on the absurd. It made little sense to me then, since what little I knew of the medical profession told me that doctors had no such preoccupation. However, as soon as I started to study the subject myself, I realised just how vital it is that the digestive tract is in perfect working order since it is the system that delivers nutrients from the food you eat into the bloodstream. I even came to think it was the medical profession that was absurd for *not* taking more interest in the subject, since without a healthy digestive tract, no matter how good your diet, you will be undernourished. The stool, its nature and frequency, gives an indication, one among many, of how well your digestive processes are functioning. As both a naturopath and a nutritionist I have since developed a particular enthusiasm for working with and correcting digestive problems. That is commonly a first step to developing good health and well-being.

The next step, running a *very* close second, is to realise how important your liver is. It is a vital part of your digestive system, but it is also much more than that. It is, if you like, the receiving and processing plant that takes the food, delivered via your digestive tract, works it over, repackages it and then ships it out to the rest of your body for use. This may be for energy production, it may be for protein building. It may be glucose to boost your blood sugar level or vitamins for your cells. It may be repackaged fats so you can deliver cholesterol to nerve and brain cells, or rearranged amino acids so you have the specific ones you need. It may be iron in a form in which it can be delivered to the bone marrow for the formation of new red blood cells. In all these actions, and hundreds more like them, the role of your liver is vital.

There is no system or part of your body that does not depend to some extent on the function of your liver or that may not be adversely affected if your liver is unhealthy, under-functioning or toxic. It is part of your immune system, it is both an exocrine (external) and endocrine (internal) gland and plays many roles in your endocrine or hormone system. On top of all that, your liver is an essential component, if not a pivotal player, in dealing with toxins in your body either breaking them down into safer substances or eliminating them from your body, either as they are, or repackaged into a safer form. If all else fails, your liver will even store toxins itself, to protect the rest of your body. However after a while, this act of generosity leads to liver damage and the rest of your body will suffer anyway.

Because of this amazing and central role that your liver plays, it becomes extremely important, in dealing with *any* health problem, to consider the state of your liver and the role it may be playing in both causing and trying to resolve the problem. Let's look at what the liver does in slightly more detail.

As a vital part of your digestive system, the liver secretes bile, without which you cannot digest fats. Faulty fat digestion can lead to associated problems with digestion in general, affecting proteins and carbohydrates as well as the fats. How can you tell whether this is happening? If you find that fatty foods disagree with you, make you feel nauseous or even bloated, this may be your problem. You may also find that your stools are pale in colour, since the colour comes from the bile pigments, or that they float or, in severe cases, that there is obvious fat in them and they stick to the pan and become difficult to flush away.

Bile also stimulates the peristaltic action of both your small and large intestine and thus helps to prevent constipation. This in turn helps to prevent a number of other intestinal problems, and to reduce the formation and absorption of several different toxins. It helps to prevent candidiasis, since having the proper movement along the intestines reduces the risk of developing an environment in which the candida mould can flourish. Bile helps to prevent allergic, or food-sensitivity, reactions within the intestinal tract and so can reduce such problems as gastritis, spastic colon and irritable bowel syndrome, all of which can be due to food sensitivities. Being constipated can lead to great pressure at the end of the colon, particularly when you try to pass a bowel motion, and this is a common cause of haemorrhoids. If all that isn't enough, by maintaining a healthy internal environment, proper peristaltic action and liver and bile function can help to reduce the risk of bowel cancer.

When you are constipated a number of toxins can build up in the digestive tract and become absorbed into the bloodstream. They then have to be dealt with by the liver in its role as a detox organ. If your liver does not deal with them your body will try to get rid of them in other ways. This may result in or aggravate skin problems as you try to eliminate them through the pores. It may put an excessive load on your kidneys. You will almost certainly find grey circles under your eyes and white fatty deposits in tissues such as the skin under your eyes and on your limbs. If all else fails you may store the toxins in your adipose tissues. These are then reluctant to break down, as the toxins would be released, and so weight loss becomes difficult. Toxins in the digestive tract can move back up the system leading to bad breath, in which case no amount of brushing your teeth and spraying with mouth deodorisers will solve the problem; it's your liver you need to work on. In fact an unhealthy liver can cause a whole range of problems related to indigestion from top to bottom.

Once bile has been produced by the liver, it is stored in the gall bladder, which then secretes it as necessary. If the liver has not done a good job, or if you have not, in your diet, supplied it with the correct raw materials, the composition of the bile may be less than optimum. This can lead to the formation of gallstones, small accretions that build up within the gall bladder, reducing both its ability to store bile and to secrete it appropriately. These stones may be made either of calcium salts, in which case they can be detected by X-rays, or of cholesterol. The latter stones are often missed, unless an ultrasound is being done for some other reason, as they may exist for a long time without causing obvious symptoms. This is unfortunate, as they can still be causing problems and, as with all health problems, the sooner you stop doing whatever caused the problem and start doing things to help fix it, the better. You will find in the Liver Detox Plan that there are many suggestions that will reduce your risk of getting gallstones and related problems.

If you have had your gall bladder removed you should still consider the suggestions given, for several reasons. First your liver still does have to produce bile and second, some people find that, almost as if in compensation for the missing bladder, pouches develop in which bile can accumulate and new stones can form. If you had your gall bladder removed but still get some of your old symptoms, then clearly your liver and digestion still need attention.

So far we have covered the digestive tract, let's now look at the role of your liver in processing the food you have eaten. Let's take one example. You eat protein, chicken protein for instance. In the digestive tract it is broken down into individual amino acids. These amino acids go to the liver where they are then recombined in a form that is suitable for the human body, into a human protein. This may be in the form of tissue proteins, needed for your muscles, organs such as your heart and kidneys, blood vessel walls and so forth. It may be proteins such as the immunoglobulins that are part of your immune system, or proteins that are part of your endocrine system, protein hormones, such as insulin that affects your blood sugar level, glucagon that affects sugar levels and energy, or calcitonin that affects bone calcium levels. Or the amino acids may be used to make amino acid derivatives that act as neuro-transmitters such as serotonin, or hormones such as thyroxine or adrenaline. Not only that, but if there is too much of one type of amino acid and not enough of another then your liver can convert the spare amounts of the first amino acid into the required amount of some types of the partially deficient ones.

Imbalances of oestrogen, progesterone and testosterone can cause a variety of problems including PMT, difficult periods and menopause, and sexual dysfunction.

Your liver also repackages the fat you eat into a variety of compounds called lipoproteins. You may have heard of 'bad cholesterol' and 'good cholesterol', although to a certain extent these are misnomers. In actual fact, what is being spoken of is these very much larger molecular complexes called lipoproteins. The cholesterol is carried in these lipoproteins and there are some (the 'bad' ones or LDLs) that carry cholesterol *to* the tissue (some of this is needed, but too much can be bad) and the others (called the 'good' ones or HDLs) that carry cholesterol *from* your tissues and get it out of your body via the gall bladder. Your liver both makes some of these proteins and repackages the cholesterol/lipoprotein complexes from one type to the other, and if it fails to do this then the LDLs, the 'bad' cholesterol-laden lipoproteins, accumulate and your heart and blood vessels are at risk.

Let's just take a moment to consider cholesterol. It has had an amazingly bad press for a substance that is needed by every single tissue in the body. It is needed for the walls of every cell in every tissue. It is needed to make bile so you can digest and absorb fats, and for the synthesis of vitamin D so you can have strong bones. You need it to make your sex hormones – without it where would the fun be? – and to make the cortisone-type hormones that are important for both your immune system and for handling stress. You also need cholesterol, in very significant amounts, for all your nerve cells and for your brain. In fact brain is the richest source of cholesterol on the menu, containing up to four times as much as an equal weight of eggs; and it is there because it is needed.

Without cholesterol, you would have indigestion and a bad liver, you couldn't handle stress or any infections, you would be a sexless, nerveless wimp with a faulty brain and no backbone, so the fact that all your cells would fall apart, leaving you a gelatinous splodge, would hardly matter. It is up to your liver to ensure that the cholesterol you eat, and the cholesterol you make within your body, perform these beneficial roles and do not get diverted into harmful activities. It is also the liver's responsibility to break down excess amounts of these various compounds when they have done their job.

A healthy liver is essential for the proper synthesis of the correct amount of this cholesterol for making good any shortfall in your diet. It is also important in that it ensures the proper transport of cholesterol through your blood *to* the tissues where it is needed and *from* the tissues where it is not needed and *could* become a problem. This also means that your liver plays a significant role in preventing the build-up of cholesterol-laden atheromas that can block your arteries and lead to heart attacks and related problems.

Another role played by the liver is that it stores glycogen, partly for its own use, but also to be able to break it down and thus release the stored glucose into the bloodstream, either when your blood sugar level falls below normal or when extra demands are made for energy, such as under stress. Hypoglycaemia (low blood sugar level) can lead to many different and varied symptoms including fatigue, shakiness, headaches, mood swings, irritability, sugar cravings and eating binges.

Stress needs no introduction – everyone has felt it and knows how it feels. If you cannot handle it, and the symptoms that result, it could pay you to treat your liver better. In relation to stress, your liver affects more than just your blood sugar level. It is capable of storing most of the B group vitamins, at least to a small extent (that's what makes liver, provided it is free of toxins, such a nutritious food and a good source of B vitamins), but this can only happen if you have fed the vitamins to your liver in the first place, either from an excellent diet or from supplements. If you didn't supply them, then all the cells in your body could be deficient. This includes vitamin B1, a deficiency of which can lead to an increased level of lactic acid in the blood, which, if not picked up immediately by the liver, can cause many symptoms that mimic a panic/anxiety attack and a heart attack combined.

Hypoglycaemia and B vitamin deficiencies can lead to fatigue. There are other causes linking your liver to fatigue. If your liver does not correctly make the proteins needed to carry iron and copper through your bloodstream and if it does not play its part in getting the iron to the bone marrow, you could suffer from anaemia. Furthermore, many fatigue problems are caused by toxins. One of the first steps, and an essential one, in dealing with ME or CFS (chronic fatigue syndrome) is a programme of detoxification. If you are tired it is definitely a sign that you need to start on the Liver Detox Plan.

A healthy liver deals with literally thousands of types of toxins every single day of your life. These include the airborne pollutants that you breathe in such as industrial pollutants from hundreds of different sources, urban ones such as car fumes, social ones such as cigarette smoke, domestic ones such as household and cosmetic chemicals, and can also come as a result of the damaging effects of radiation and electromagnetic fields (even sitting in front of the television can cause problems). They include the thousands of toxic chemicals that can be in your food as a result of agricultural processes, food processes and preserving, from the water supply or by accident. They also come from the substances applied to your skin, from drugs (social or medical), medications and a number of other miscellaneous sources. Furthermore, a number of toxic substances are made in your body as you metabolise used tissues and materials such as hormones that have done their job.

Your liver either gets rid of these toxins directly, via your gall bladder in bile and through the digestive tract, or it converts them to safer compounds, i.e. the conversion of ammonia (from proteins) to urea, or else it breaks them down altogether. Ammonia is so unsafe that, once in the brain, it can cause severe symptoms, leading eventually to coma and death. The efficient processing of toxins can protect you from a variety of degenerative diseases including heart disease, diabetes and arthritis, and can reduce your risk of getting cancer. This on its own should encourage you to follow the Liver Detox Plan.

Your liver repackages various other nutrients, including some of the vitamins, such as vitamin A and E, and some minerals, such as iron and copper, as we have seen. If this repackaging is not completed efficiently, you may, for example, experience both vitamin A deficiency signs in the surrounding tissues and vitamin A toxicity signs as it accumulates in the liver. The liver stores B vitamins needed for energy, particularly B12, of which it can store several weeks' supply.

Your liver is involved in your immune system and helps to protect you from infections. This results from the action of special liver cells called Kupffer cells that help to get rid of toxins. If these Kupffer cells are not healthy, this aspect of your immune system does not function. Furthermore, if your liver does not get rid of old hormones, your levels of white blood cells and antibodies will fall below normal. (The white cells are the ones that scavenge foreign invaders and toxins, and your antibodies are the special proteins that fight the individual antigens or invaders from outside.)

An extension of this relationship between your liver and your immune system is the relationship between a healthy liver and allergic reactions. For many reasons, if your liver is not healthy you will be allergy prone and this can lead to a whole range of symptoms from acne to asthma, from migraines to arthritis, from sinus problems and catarrh to hay fever and watering eyes, from mood swings and behavioural problems to candidiasis and psychiatric problems and many more.

Whether you get your vitamin D from your diet, or make it yourself by the action of sunlight on your skin, your liver is necessary for the ultimate activity of this vitamin since it is converted into its active form in the liver. This means that you could find that a faulty liver, rather than a deficiency of calcium or vitamin D, is responsible for calcium deficiency, which may eventually lead to osteoporosis.

Another problem that may be linked to a malfunctioning liver is that of being overweight. If your liver cannot or does not deal with toxins, and since many of them are fat-soluble, it may store them in your adipose tissues – those rolls and bulges all over your body. Once stored in these tissues, the toxins are relatively harmless. However if that tissue was to be broken down, they would be released and could cause you harm. So, as a self-defence mechanism, your body may then refuse to break down these adipose tissues even when you reduce the amount you eat and need the fat the tissues contain for energy. This would then mean that dieting would leave you not only frustrated but exhausted. If this seems familiar, then the Liver Detox Plan is a must. Once you have been on it for a few days or a few weeks (depending on your own particular metabolisms and level of toxins) you could suddenly find that any excess weight you may be carrying starts to come off with very little effort.

A toxic liver can also contribute to cravings, such as sugar cravings or a craving for chocolate or alcohol; once you improve the state of your liver it will be so much easier to stick to a healthy eating programme. This can improve not only your health, but also your weight, since you will no longer feel like going on those sugar or alcohol binges.

As if all that isn't enough, your liver is also important for your moods and emotional state and for your memory and your ability to think and concentrate clearly. Furthermore, an unhealthy liver, by its negative effect on your energy levels, can leave you too tired to bother, if not out and out exhausted. In this and many other ways the functioning of your liver will affect your emotions, attitude, mood and thinking.

What else can harm your liver? Do you drink alcohol? This is damaging in itself, it is also converted into other toxic compounds that contribute to many of the hangover symptoms, and it further stresses and damages your liver. Do you love fats, cream, mayonnaise, chocolate, coffee? Do you smoke cigarettes or take any drugs, social, recreational or medical? Do you eat late at night and then go to bed before the meal is digested? There are so many things that people do, without even thinking, that damage the liver that it is a wonder it serves you as well as it does. The exciting thing is that once you accept that you have *chosen* to do these things you will also realise that you are free to choose *not* to do these things. It is up to you. *You* are in control.

Summary

With all this in mind, think what an awesome task you liver has, how many different roles it has to play and the hundreds, if not thousands, of ways it can affect the rest of your body and its function. Think what can happen if your liver fails to do its job properly. You could have indigestion, atherosclerosis, diabetes, hormone imbalances, PMS, period or menopausal problems or headaches and migraines. You could develop allergies, leading to a vast range of symptoms ranging from eczema to asthma, migraines to arthritis, sinusitis to hives, behavioural problems, mood swings and mental confusion. You could experience blood sugar imbalances with all the many associated problems, and hundreds of different vitamin and mineral deficiency signs. You would doubtless feel tired, for many different reasons, have poor skin and hair health. You could be an overweight but persistent, yo-yo and unsuccessful dieter, and to cap it off your risk of cancer would be greatly increased. If you think that that sounds like a lot, it isn't even the whole story, the liver does so many things it is difficult to list them all.

You may be wondering by now how well your own liver is functioning. Before you rush off to the doctor for a liver function test, stop. It is possible to have normal blood tests for a long time after your liver is subtly and in many different ways, beginning to fail to do its job efficiently and successfully. Only when your liver is very seriously sick will these blood tests actually show that there is a problem. Long before that your liver may have been letting you down, and letting you down badly. You may have many health problems and have made many attempts to correct the situation but without treating your liver your efforts could have been wasted.

If this introduction has already set you thinking, and you would like to start right away to make the changes that will benefit your liver, then do so. However since it is generally useful to know why you are doing things and to know which things in particular are important for you to do, I do recommend reading Section 2. Furthermore, when the going gets tough, when you feel that 'surely it can't matter' if you have another cigarette, cup of coffee or a drink for the road, when the desserts look tempting, the cream and other fats are irresistible and you'd rather use household chemicals than clean the old-fashioned way or prefer to spread pesticides instead of weeding the garden, read it again. There's nothing like being reminded of the facts to keep the importance of what you are doing in the forefront of your mind.

Happy reading and good health.

Part II

The Liver Detox Plan

As a starting-point, your liver's ability to function and to rebuild and repair itself is absolutely dependent on the quality of the food, the raw materials, you consume. Your liver *cannot* be better than the quality of the food and nutrients you give it. It can be worse, depending on what else you do to it. Eating badly and expecting to have a fully healthy liver is like expecting to build a beautiful home with faulty bricks. With faulty bricks you *cannot* have a secure house, no matter how good the architect or how fine the location.

With good bricks you *can* have a fine house, but if the architect is poor it may still not be such a good house. In the same way, even if you *do* eat all the foods and nutrients you need, if you then fail to improve your lifestyle, your liver may still not be perfect. So, it is important to improve your nutrient intake *and* reduce your toxic load and harmful habits.

What you eat and the supplements you take are of paramount importance to the liver in at least four ways:

1. **The liver's own needs:** your liver, like any other organ in your body, needs nutrients for its own health and protection from harm, so give it foods that can deliver these nutrients and avoid giving it substances that are harmful or damaging to it.

2. **Its role in digestion:** your liver then has to process the food you eat. Great demands are made on it during the digestive process, so be kind and give it foods it can digest readily rather than those with which it has to struggle.

3. **Its ability to deliver suitable substances to the rest of your body:** thirdly your liver has special needs to enable it to send out nutrients to the rest of your body, either in an absorbed form or suitably transformed into other compounds. This latter is particularly important as otherwise you may eat things needed by other tissues, but find that your liver cannot do its intermediate job and the benefit is negligible. So give it what it needs to do this job too.

4. **Its role in detoxification:** your liver has particular needs, unique to its essential role in dealing with a lot of the toxins you either take on board or produce within your own body.

Your liver is a very clever organ, but it cannot stop your hand pouring that additional whiskey, picking up the cream jug or unwrapping yet another chocolate bar, and it cannot force you to prepare the salad, take the supplements or drink the dandelion coffee. In this somewhat helpless capacity all it can do is try to cope, the best it can, with what you send down the tube. For your own sake, be kind to it.

There are few people who haven't already done harm to their liver. Unless you have led an extraordinary life, you probably aren't one of them. However the same technology and growth in our understanding of our world and our bodies that have brought so many adverse effects, have also given us the understanding and the technology to create a variety of beneficial nutritional supplements that can help you to repair and, in time, avoid, some of the damage that has been inflicted. In the Liver Detox Plan you will learn about a range of substances you can take that are particularly therapeutic and beneficial to your liver. At least initially, it is important that you take these to help restore your liver to better health. Ideally, many of them should also have a role to play in the prevention of possible future problems. However many people do not want to take too many supplements on an ongoing basis, so at the end of the programme you will find a description of a basic and minimal maintenance supplement programme, together with a maintenance diet. The combination of the two should help to keep the improved health and well-being you develop during the Liver Detox Plan.

There is one problem with preventive healthcare, and it is important that you realise this – you never know what you have prevented. You cannot know, once you start on the Liver Detox Plan, and when, at some time in the future you begin to wonder if it was all really necessary, how well, or how ill, you might have been had you not made the effort. Let me assure you that, in over 20 years of advising people in this way, the benefits I have seen have been significant. Many times people have responded well. Others have responded and then, some years later, let things slide, thinking they have done all they need, only to then get sick again, come back and start the process all over again. Fortunately they often find that they are able to recover yet again, though perhaps not as well as the first time, since damage has been done along the way. There are also times when people find that they have allowed the damage to progress too far and they cannot regain their earlier health, but at least they can prevent or slow down any further damage. My best advice is, start now and promise yourself you will maintain the programme.

Dietary Factors

Your body, and therefore your liver, needs, in addition to fresh air and pure water, the three major food categories, namely proteins, fats and carbohydrates, plus the minor nutrients, needed in relatively small, but critically important amounts, and generally grouped together as vitamins and minerals.

Vitamins are small organic molecules; minerals, in this context, are single elements. In general they are both needed in small quantities because they are not used up during the chemical reactions in which they are involved. Instead they act as assistants, or coenzymes – it's a bit like a policeman helping a large number of people cross a road after some big event. At the end of the stint on duty there are still the same number of police as there were at the start, but hundreds or even thousands more people have been able to cross safely than would have been possible if they had to wait for gaps in the traffic.

In addition to acting as coenzymes, vitamins and minerals perform other roles. Obvious examples include the calcium and other minerals that make up your bones and the iron in your red blood cells. This is why you need these nutrients in greater amounts than those that are purely coenzymes.

You may be wondering why, if the coenzyme vitamins and minerals are not used up, you need to keep taking them. This is because they do, eventually, either break down or get lost in the urine, sweat or stools. It is also true that you can either function on economy rations or in luxury. If you take small amounts of all the nutrients you may survive but at below optimum levels. If you take generous quantities you may be much healthier, happier and more energetic. The choice is, of course, yours.

Before we describe these trace nutrients further, let's look at the three main food components.

Carbohydrate Foods

The Different Types

Foods rich in carbohydrates include sugars, grains, fruits, vegetables, and legumes. Legumes also contain significant amounts of protein, and even the grains do contain protein that, because of the quantity of grains generally eaten, contribute significantly to the total protein content of the diet.

There are several different types of carbohydrates. They range from the simple sugars in fruits, honey and table sugar, through the large complex carbohydrates such as the starches in vegetables and grains, to the non-digestible carbohydrates, commonly, though inaccurately, called fibre. You need generous amounts of fibre and complex carbohydrates in your diet, but no sugar.

Out Go the Sugars

Much though you may enjoy sugar, honey, various syrups and the foods in which they play a leading role, you have absolutely no nutritional need for sugar whatsoever, even though you may have a sweet tooth. True, it may give you energy, but not much, and not in the long term since it lacks the B vitamins and minerals that have to work with the sugar to release its energy. Sugar may also roller-coaster you into 'energy highs' followed by 'energy dumps', as your blood sugar falls again. Furthermore, if you eat sugar your liver will have to work harder and manipulate its glycogen stores more than normal to aid the pancreas and other glands that secrete the hormones needed in the battle to maintain normal blood sugar levels.

The Important Whole Grains

The starches from grains can come either 'refined' (e.g. white flour and white rice) or 'unrefined' (e.g. wholemeal flour and brown rice). Your liver will not benefit greatly from refined carbohydrates since, like sugar, they provide the calories without all the trace nutrients, so they provide neither the fibre needed for your digestive tract nor all the vitamins and minerals need for your liver and the rest of your body. They can, on the other hand, contribute to the hypoglycaemic energy slump so often experienced in the afternoon or an hour or two after eating. All these foods should go out of your diet and out of your kitchen!

Instead, what you need are foods rich in the unrefined, complex carbohydrates that deliver the starch that gives you energy as well as the protein, fibre, vitamins and trace minerals necessary for the many functions your liver has to perform. Foods rich in these unrefined carbohydrates include porridge oats, brown rice, wholemeal flour and products made from it, including wholemeal pasta and wholemeal bread. Include other grains as well, such as rye and barley and products made from or with them, such as rye bread and barley in soups. All these foods supply valuable nutrients including fibre, the B vitamins, coenzyme Q10, vitamin E and a variety of minerals including copper, chromium, iron, magnesium, manganese, molybdenum and zinc.

These unrefined complex carbohydrates are broken down in the digestive tract much more slowly than their refined counterparts, so their nutrients are delivered slowly into the bloodstream, as is the glucose that comes from the gradual breakdown of the starch. As a result your blood sugar level is kept relatively constant, the hypoglycaemic slumps are avoided and liver glycogen can build up. You should incorporate a number of these wholegrain products into your programme, though you may find you are being asked to eat more vegetables and fewer grains than you have done in the past.

Don'ts

Do not eat sugar, honey or other refined carbohydrates. If you want something sweet, eat fresh fruit. If you eat dried fruit make sure it is sulphur-free, as the sulphur compounds damage several of the B vitamins. This will probably mean the dried fruit is dark in colour, but it will still be tasty. Dried fruit such as dates and figs are generally sprayed with pesticides that irritate the intestinal tract (hence their reputation as laxatives), so ideally ask not only for organically grown dried fruit but for fruit that also states it has not been sprayed. As part of the Liver Detox Plan you are going to be taking a supplement of B vitamins and this, in time, will reduce your craving for any other sugar in your diet.

Fruit and Vegetables

Vegetables are the major source of vitamins and minerals in your diet, when measured on the basis of the amount you get for the number of calories they provide. In other words they are extremely nutrient-dense foods. For every 100 calories you take in you will, in general, get more trace nutrients and more vitamins and minerals, from them than from most other foods. That is a sweeping statement and, like all sweeping statements, there are exceptions to it. An egg, for instance, is a highly-nutrient dense food. However, in view of the lowly place most people accord to vegetables in their diet, it is worth stating their benefits loudly and strongly. They are particularly important for your liver and they are particularly important on any detox programme.

Fruit is somewhat less nutrient dense, being richer in fruit sugars and containing fewer trace nutrients. However it contains some nutrients, like vitamin C, the bioflavonoids and pycnogenols or OPCs, that are essential for your health and for a safe detox programme.

Vegetables and fruit also have an alkalising effect on the body, due to their high content of trace minerals, regardless of whether or not they contain acids themselves. This is important because fats, proteins and complex carbohydrates all produce carbon dioxide and hence carbonic acid when they break down. Fruit and vegetables help to maintain balance.

For these reasons fruit and vegetables should make up a large part of your diet – almost certainly a larger part than they play at present. Time and time again patients tell me that they eat lots of fruit and vegetables. 'Lots' is a subjective amount and open to individual interpretation. While it is true that you may eat several vegetables at one meal in the day, usually dinner, it is unlikely that you eat them in significant quantities at *all* meals in the day. Nor is it likely that they make up a major proportion of your snacks – yet they should.

Ideally, as we shall see, you should incorporate fruit generously into your breakfast (Original Muesli, Fruit Salad and Yoghurt, see recipes) or you should include some vegetables (vegetable omelettes, scrambled eggs with tomatoes, peppers and onions). At lunchtime choose a salad or some other vegetable dish. When you want a snack have a piece of fruit, or perhaps some vegetable sticks (Carrot Sticks with Humus, etc). Dinner can then include the traditional meat, potatoes and two (or three) veg with fruit to follow (Fruit Salad recipes and variations).

That is not what you have been doing? I thought not. Yet this programme can make a wonderful difference to your liver. Not only does it remove from your diet those fatty, sugary, liver- and artery-clogging foods that put a load on your liver, but it also gives your liver many of the vital nutrients it needs.

While vegetables in general are beneficial, there are some that are particularly important for your liver, either directly by their effect on the liver, or indirectly, by taking over some of the work your liver would otherwise have to do. Only selected vegetables have been included in the table below, however you should not underestimate the others. Vegetables that are strongly coloured, such as carrots, pumpkins and dark-leaved vegetables, provide many beneficial nutrients including the carotenes that help prevent cancer. Most fruit and leaves are rich in vitamin C and most leaves are rich in folic acid. It may surprise you to know that many vegetables, particularly those above ground, will also give you more calcium than milk (on the basis of more calcium for your calories) and that they do this without giving you the phosphorous that is found in milk (an excess of which can actually increase your loss of calcium in the urine) and at the same time providing many other minerals as well.

Table 1: **Vegetables that are particularly good for your liver**

Alfalfa sprouts: alkalising and rich in minerals. Even if you live in a flat you can grow them for yourself.

Artichoke, globe: a member of the thistle family, this has a history of helping to reduce blood levels of fats and cholesterol via its action on the liver, where it stimulates the production and excretion of bile and reduces the liver's synthesis of cholesterol. Helps to reduce fatty livers, improves the liver's detoxification capacity and helps to protect the liver and improve its capacity for repair and regeneration. It contains inulin *(see Jerusalem artichoke)*.

Bean and seed sprouts: like alfalfa sprouts, you can grow these, fresh, for yourself. Buy organic beans and seeds and grow them like mustard and cress, keeping them well watered and washed so mould doesn't form. If you need more details, there are many books that can help. Sprout the different legumes such as soy beans and chick peas, and seeds such as sunflower seeds.

Beetroot: has a history of protecting the liver and reducing the risk of cancer.

Broccoli: helps the liver to excrete oestrogen and thus reduces the risk of breast cancer.

Brussels sprouts: similar actions to cabbage and broccoli.

Cabbage: contains substances that improve antioxidant and detoxification activity and increase oestrogen metabolism, all functions of the liver; can also help in the treatment of stomach ulcers.

Collards and kale: these are also members of the cabbage family and are packed full of nutrients including carotenes, vitamin C and minerals, including more calcium than milk.

Dandelion: is normally thought of as a weed and a pest. However it is an excellent liver remedy *(see under Herbs)*. It has also been shown to help dieters to lose weight, possibly through its detox effect as well as its effect on the kidneys and its diuretic action. The leaves can be added to salad or cooked with other greens. The root is generally roasted, ground and made into a coffee. This is available in most health food shops in two forms, either in the instant form mixed with lactose (milk sugar) or as a roasted and ground root which needs to be simmered for 20 minutes and strained before it is ready to drink. This is nutritionally better, but less convenient. If it is too much trouble to simmer your own, use the instant variety rather than regular coffee, except during the six weeks of the Liver Detox Plan itself, when you should make the effort to use the ground root.

Fennel: helps to improve digestion, tone the digestive tract and prevent flatulence and colic. By improving normal digestion it reduces the work the liver has to do and improves nutrient absorption.

Garlic: has possibly more benefits than any other vegetable or culinary herb and you will find it in many of the recipes. It is well known for its beneficial effect on the immune system, being used in the treatment of colds and influenza. It is a natural antibiotic, being both antibacterial and antiviral; it is also useful in the treatment of parasites and worms, is effective against moulds and in the treatment of candida, and is thought to help protect against cancer. Perhaps less known is its powerful action in lowering the level of cholesterol, lowering the glucose level when abnormally high (as in diabetes) and reducing high blood pressure. It is of still further value to your heart in that it reduces the risk of unwanted blood clots. Garlic contains sulphur groups that complex with toxic metals, such as mercury, thus helping the detoxification action of the liver. In these ways it works with the liver and can reduce the work of the liver.

Jerusalem artichoke: both globe and Jerusalem artichoke contain inulin. This is a complex carbohydrate that is not broken down by the body, does not produce energy, and so the artichoke is effectively low in calories. The leaves contain compounds (caffeylquinic acids) that are protective, promote liver regeneration and aid the normal flow of bile. The artichoke must be fresh, otherwise the inulin breaks down, in the plant, into sugars. Inulin nourishes the beneficial bacteria in the intestines, particularly bifidobacteria which is essential to a healthy digestive tract.

Leeks: act similarly to onions, but you need more to get the same effect.

Onions: are rich in many nutrients, including bioflavonoids and calcium. In the same family as garlic, they also contain sulphur compounds that help in detox programmes, help to normalise the blood cholesterol level, reduce the risk of unwanted blood clots and normalise blood sugar levels, possibly by protecting insulin and possibly by increasing the liver's metabolism of glucose. There is also evidence that onions help to reduce tumour growth.

Parsley: is rich in carotenoids, vitamin C and bioflavonoids, plus many trace minerals. Its chlorophyll can help to reduce the odour of other foods, such as garlic. Parsley is a mild diuretic and can help reduce fluid retention and high blood pressure.

Radish: another vegetable that is thought to help the liver directly, it also stimulates digestion.

Turnip: a member of the cabbage family *(see above)*. The leaves should be eaten as well as the root.

Watercress: is rich in beta-carotene and sulphur, both of which are good for the liver. Use it both in and to decorate salads.

Table 2: **Fruits that are good for your liver**

Apple and pears: apples and pears are a good source of pectin, a soluble form of fibre that can help prevent constipation and lower blood cholesterol. Ironically it can also help prevent diarrhoea: a good remedy is to grate an apple or pear, including the skin, let it go brown and then eat it. The pectin also combines with toxins in the gut. Apples contain compounds that help prevent cancer.

Apricot: a good source of carotenes and some trace minerals.

Avocado: a useful source of the essential fatty acid and linoleic acid, also contains vitamins in the B group, vitamin E and potassium.

Banana: the fruit people eat who don't really like fruit! High in starch and sugars, also in potassium. Bananas have soothed some cases of ulcers in the digestive tract.

Berries: there are many different berries, including blackberries, blueberries, raspberries and strawberries. In general, the darker they are, the more nutrients they contain, such as bioflavonoids and the newly recognised proanthocyanidins or OPCs, plus carotenes and vitamin C.

Cranberries: beneficial to the kidneys, they acidify the urine, inhibit E. coli and improve detoxification; useful in the treatment of cystitis.

Grapefruit: slows down Step 1 of a detox programme and thus helps to reduce possible reactions; encourages the elimination of old red blood cells; contains pectin (particularly the edible solids), which helps to lower blood cholesterol.

Grapes: the grape diet was commonly recognised as a detox programme, 10 or 20 years ago, as was a grape juice fast. Grapes contain proanthocyanidins, powerful antioxidants that help the detox programme and help prevent atherosclerosis.

Lemons: the juice and the white pith of lemons contain limonen, which helps to dissolve gallstones. They also contain pectin and vitamin C.

Oranges: good sources of vitamin C and pectin.

Papaya: aids digestion (papain is a protein-splitting enzyme), contains antioxidants.

Pineapple: aids digestion (bromelain is a protein-splitting enzyme).

Watermelon: a diuretic, useful in detox.

Keep in mind that toxins may be lurking on and in the fruit and vegetables you buy, so buy organically grown vegetables and fruit whenever you can. You can augment these too, by growing them yourself. This can be done no matter how small your garden. Follow the Continental habit of growing them in the front garden as well as the back, and mix them in with your flowers. Even if you have no garden, grow them on your balcony, on the window-ledge or in pots. If you set your mind to it you will be surprised at just how many tomatoes you can grow on a balcony, how many baby lettuces, carrots and radishes you can grow in window boxes and how many herbs you can grow in lieu of house plants, in pots distributed near your windows. If you have them in pots in your kitchen, you will find frequent uses for them.

Fibre is Essential

Fibre is essential to any detox programme. Strictly speaking fibre is not fibre – in most cases it is not even fibrous (celery strands excepted). Instead it may be a fine powder, or it may even, when combined with the fluids in your digestive tract, produce a jelly. So a better name for it is 'non-digestible carbohydrate'.

Because such substances are not digested or broken down in the small intestine they enter the colon, where they feed the beneficial bacteria there and add bulk to the stool by absorbing water and swelling up. So fibre improves your intestinal environment, helps to prevent the flatulence and bloating that can occur when the wrong type of organisms are present, and helps to prevent constipation. Fibre also helps in the detox programme by absorbing many of the toxins in the digestive tract, in the stomach, small intestine and colon. For instance, it can combine with some of the toxic trace metals. It can also combine with steroids such as cholesterol and the products of 'waste' hormones, and ensure that they are carried out in the stool rather than reabsorbed back into the bloodstream.

You will hear fibre spoken of as 'soluble' and 'insoluble'. Don't worry too much about the details. It simply means, in effect, that some are mucilaginous and protect the lining of the digestive tract, some are soft bulking agents, others are more active in preventing constipation and some are particularly good at combining with toxins. Since many foods contain a combination of several different types of fibre, the best thing to do is to consider the overall fibre-rich foods, as listed below, for specific problems, but in general to include generous amounts of a variety of different fibre-rich foods in your diet.

The prime benefits of fibre are to the health and function of your digestive system and the positive consequences that flow on from that. They give a feeling of fullness, especially if taken with plenty of fluid, and so can help you if you are also trying to diet and lose weight, particularly if taken shortly before a meal, and they help you to lower your blood cholesterol level and so improve circulation.

Vegetable Fibre

The best type of fibre is that found in fruit and vegetables, rather than that in grains. Why? Possibly because for millions of years the diet of humans and their forebears was built around fruit and vegetables and they adapted to the fibre in them. It is only in the last 10,000 years that grains have come to play a role in our diet and, in the evolutionary scheme of things, this is a very tiny length of time indeed. While we have evolved and adapted to vegetable fibres, we have not, it seems, yet fully adapted to grain fibre.

The need for fibre is a further reason, in addition to those given above, to include generous amounts of vegetables and fruit in your diet several times a day. Remember that on the whole vegetables have considerably more fibre than fruit, but that fruit does also contribute some fibre to your diet, not all of it obvious, such as the pectin in apples, pears and citrus fruit.

Grain Fibre

After fruit and vegetables the next best type of fibre is that found in whole grains, but it is best eaten combined with the whole grain, as in wholemeal flour or brown rice, rather than as the bran on its own. Some people find that when, for instance, they use wheat bran or oat bran to help deal with their constipation, they actually get even more constipated or develop abdominal pains. In part this may be because they have not drunk sufficient water with the fibre, but this doesn't always explain the symptoms. The same people may feel fine when they eat the whole grains, however, we also know that the grains, particularly wheat, are among the most common allergens. If you have an unsuspected allergy or sensitivity to wheat and try to use wheat bran to cure your constipation, this may be counter productive. This should not put you off grain fibres, however, simply encourage you to give vegetable fibre the importance it deserves and to eat whole grains rather than refined ones.

Grain fibre occurs mainly in the bran or outside skin of each grain which also contains trace minerals and B vitamins. Use wholemeal flour instead of white flour, wholemeal bread instead of white bread, wholemeal pasta instead of pasta made with white flour, brown rice instead of white rice, etc., as already mentioned. Rolled or porridge oats still have their bran, so does rye in the form in which it is commonly sold.

Some people argue against eating bran, saying that it contains phytic acid and that combines with minerals, inhibiting their absorption. This may be true, but the minerals are in the bran, rather than in the rest of the grain, so if you don't eat the bran you won't get those minerals any-way, and the fibre in the bran is important. What's more, if you take an evolutionary perspective we did eat the bran, right up until very recent times, and we managed very well on it.

Legume Fibre

Legumes, such as lentils, red kidney beans, soy beans, chick peas and other beans, usually sold either dried or in tins, contain considerable amounts of fibre. This group also includes peanuts, which are actually beans, not nuts. However peanuts are inadvisable in that they can con-tain an invisible mould called aflotoxin that can cause cancer. Legumes are an excellent source of low-fat protein, complex carbohydrates and fibre, as well as trace nutrients. There is, however, one warning in regard to legumes. If your digestion is poor or your liver really overloaded, you may find these foods difficult to digest. Their digestion depends upon an enzyme from your pancreas called trypsin and the legumes contain a substance that reduces the effectiveness of this enzyme. Peanuts are the worst in this regard, followed by soy beans, then other beans and finally lentils. The ultimate test is yourself. If you do not get wind, then you can digest them. Even if you have trouble digesting them you should be able to digest altered soy products such as tofu and soy milk.

Specific Fibre Sources

To find out what the following substances do when inside your intestines you can try a simple experiment. Put a small quantity, say a tablespoon, in a tall glass, add water at blood heat, stir and then watch what happens.

Linseeds

Linseeds can be used in two ways and for two different reasons. They will combine with water in the digestive tract, swell up and form a jelly that helps propel the food and waste material along the digestive tract and prevent constipation. If, however, you chew them thoroughly (diffi-cult to do as they are small) or grind them into a flour and then eat them immediately, the essential fatty acids that they contain can be absorbed and will benefit your liver and your cardiovascular system and other tissues as well.

Pectin

Pectin is the substance often sold for the purpose of making jams and marmalade set. It is found in fruit such as apples and pears and in citrus fruit. By a similar action to the one it has in jam, combining with water in your gut, it can help to prevent constipation and can also lower blood cholesterol levels. It should be eaten as part of the fruit. There is more in the solid edible parts of citrus fruit than in the juice.

Psyllium Hulls

Look for ground or powdered psyllium hulls. These hulls come from the husk of the seed (like bran). They contain soluble fibre and mucilaginous compounds that help to prevent constipation. They also absorb toxins and help to eliminate them from the digestive tract. These toxins include the chemicals produced by the mould candida albicans and it can also help to remove candida organisms themselves. Since candidiasis is a common, and often unsuspected, problem, and since it leads to the production of a number of toxins, all of which add to the toxic load on the liver, psyllium will play a significant role in the Liver Detox Plan.

Slippery Elm

Slippery elm is the powdered inner bark of the elm tree. It is a very gentle form of non-digestible carbohydrate and very rich in mucilaginous components. One to two teaspoonfuls, taken morning and night, will line the walls of the stomach and intestine and protect them if there is any erosion or damage, such as is found in ulcers or incipient ulcers, gastritis, ileitis or colitis. It also provides soft bulk to the stool to help remove toxins and gently prevent constipation.

Fats

The different types of fats and what they do are covered in Section 2, so only a few brief comments are given here. There are saturated fats, unsaturated fats and polyunsaturated fats. The polyunsaturated ones have had a few years of popularity, however they are also polyunstable, with an increased risk of going rancid or being oxidised, at each point of unsaturation, and being converted into toxins, including carcinogens, unless fully protected by antioxidants. For this reason, olive oil, a slightly unsaturated oil, has many health benefits to offer over either the more saturated butter and animal fats or the polyunsaturated vegetable oils. Buy the best quality virgin olive oil that you can find.

If you eat butter, buy unsalted butter and make sure it is absolutely fresh. If there is any discoloration of the surface (rancidity), scrape it off and eat only the butter that is below this surface. You should aim to keep the total amount of saturated fats in your diet (such as butter and most animal fats) to a minimum. However you do need some fats in your diet to supply the essential fatty acids. These are vital for your health and needed by every cell in your body, but, since you cannot make them it is also essential that they come from your diet. Oil-rich fish such as sardines, salmon and mackerel are an excellent source. EFAs are also obtainable from pure linseed oil. Available in some health food shops they are made from organic linseeds and stored so that they are protected from oxidation. Better still, eat the freshly ground linseeds. Other excellent sources include evening primrose oil and borage oil. Other seeds that are rich in the important fatty acids are sunflower seeds and sesame seeds (chew them well). Eat avocado pears and fresh olives, and eat nuts, but they should be raw, not either plain roasted or salted (and not peanuts). You will also get some oil from the beans that you eat, such as soy beans.

These fats and oils will supply you with the essential fatty acids. They will also stimulate the gall bladder, and thus the flow of bile. This is healthy and prevents stasis and the risk of gallstones. (However a very high-fat diet puts too much of a load on the liver's ability to produce bile.) It is now generally thought that about 35 per cent of the calories in your diet should come from fats. Most people eat between 40 and 50 per cent as fat so it is probable that to achieve the optimum diet you will have to reduce the amount of fat you are eating significantly. Since much of the fat you eat is 'hidden', and since fats provide more than twice as many calories per gram as carbohydrates or proteins, you may be unaware of your actual total intake.

Some types of fat are to be avoided at all costs. These include the hydrogenated fats, and the trans fatty acids they can contain, which are harmful in many ways. This means avoiding margarines and all similar spreads. Read the labels carefully and look for a guarantee that the products and their ingredients have not been hydrogenated. You should also avoid foods that have been fried at a high temperature, such as chips and other deep-fat fried foods as these can contained hydrogenated fats. Rancid fats should also be avoided, hence the instruction above regarding butter. Heating fats to smoking heat can cause serious harm to them, and to you if you consume them.

Keep in mind that cholesterol is an important nutrient, and not simply the dangerous compound you have been led to believe, so do include eggs in your diet. They are actually an excellent source of many different nutrients. If you are concerned about your cholesterol level you should keep your total fat intake down, increase your intake of fibre and increase your intake of lecithin and the B group vitamins, particularly vitamin B6.

Lecithin

The lecithins, more commonly referred to in the singular, lecithin, are a vitally important group of fats. Lecithin is an emulsifying agent that has many benefits in the body, improving fat digestion, liver and gall bladder function and the metabolism of cholesterol. It is needed in the walls of all your cells, and in your brain and nervous tissues. You can make lecithin in your own body, provided you have sufficient quantities of the essential fatty acids, methionine, vitamin B6, choline and several other nutrients, but if your liver is under stress it makes sense to ensure there is a generous amount in your diet.

Lecithin is in eggs because of its importance to the developing embryo, so this is another good reason to include eggs in the diet. It can also be extracted from soy beans and you can buy it as granules or in capsule or tablet form. The granules have a taste that is slightly similar to that of butter and about as strong. They can be sprinkled over food, on salads, or stirred into a liquid, such as fruit juice. However, because lecithin contains unsaturated and polyunsaturated fats and because these can go rancid, it is important that it is fresh. Buy carefully, looking at the date, and buy small quantities. Once the packet is opened make sure you keep the lecithin in an airtight container and eat it quickly. Aim to have about a tablespoon a day. If you prefer to take a supplement choose an oil-filled capsule rather than a tablet and take three capsules daily, of 1,000 to 1,200 mg.

The best way to summarise your fat intake is to say that it is the quality that is all important, even more so than the total amount. As regards the amount, you should probably reduce your intake slightly, but not as excessively as some people have been recommending, say to about 35 per cent of your calories, sufficient, among other things, to provide normal stimulation for your gall bladder. Reduce your intake of the fully saturated fats and the very unsaturated ones. Totally avoid hydrogenated fats (margarine) and those heated to a high temperature (fried foods) and rancid fats and, where possible, eat them as they occur naturally, in nuts, seeds, avocado pears, etc. The same is true of cholesterol. The quality is more important than the amount. Avoid overcooked cholesterol (hard-fried eggs) and eat plenty of lecithin and vitamin B6.

Protein

Some naturopaths, natural therapists or enthusiastic consumers will recommend such regimes as fasting, drinking only fruit juices, living on fruit and vegetables, or on a diet of brown rice. These regimes may seem to be cleansing but they have a major failing. They do not contain protein (or, in the case of rice, sufficient protein) and this is a serious flaw. When your diet is lacking in sufficient protein your body starts to draw on the protein of your liver, to its detriment. So it is important that you have adequate protein both on the detox regime and on your future maintenance diet.

At the start of the Liver Detox Plan this protein will come from fish as this is lower in fat than meat. You will be avoiding eggs and dairy products to begin with but they will come in, progressively, later. Legume protein, as explained above, may be difficult to digest and it too has to wait until later in the programme to be included. You may also be able to purchase special dietary food powders, with readily digestible protein, that are dairy and soy free and don't contain sugar or flavourings; you can include these as well.

In general, the protein should come from a variety of sources and, unless you are a vegetarian or vegan, should include both plant and animal protein. Avoid protein foods that are also rich in fats, such as streaky bacon and high-fat cuts of meat. Do choose fish several times a week, particularly the oily fishes as they contain linolenic acid, an essential fatty acid that leads to the formation of the protective PG3 group of prostaglandins. Legumes, the dried peas and beans, are good sources of vegetable protein, and combine well with the protein in grains. The total amount in grains may be small (approximately 6 to 14 per cent) but the quality, particularly the quality of rice protein, is good.

Choose protein foods with a minimum amount of processing and avoid smoked foods or ones to which nitrates have been added. This means avoiding sausages, nearly all of which are high in fat and many of which are smoked. Avoid frankfurters which are high in fat, blood and chemicals and low in protein. As with all foods the aim should be to buy the food as close as possible to the form in which it is grown or lives. This means being able to see the form of the flesh, the shape of the chicken breast, fillet of fish or leg of lamb, rather than buying an amorphous meat ball, with uncertain contents.

Amino Acids

Protein is made up of dozens, often hundreds, of amino acids. Up to 20 different ones are involved, and some of these also play roles as individuals. These may be involved in the brain, as messenger molecules, as hormones. Certain amino acids are very specifically involved with the liver and its functions.

Cysteine

Three amino acids, cysteine, methionine and taurine, contain sulphur and this is very important for the detoxifying actions of the liver for several reasons. A large amount of damage is done by toxins that cause oxidation of important compounds and tissues, often as a result of the production of free radicals. You need lots of antioxidants to help protect you from the damage these unstable and destructive parts of molecules can do.

One important antioxidant is cysteine. It leads to increased levels of another antioxidant called glutathione. Cysteine and glutathione improve detoxification and protect against cell death caused by toxins or oxidation. Thus it both protects the liver and enables the liver to protect the rest of the body. Either cysteine or methionine is required for the synthesis of taurine which, in turn is needed for the production of bile salts.

Methionine

Methionine is an essential amino acid. It is also a component of SAM (S-adenosylmethionine), probably the most important single substance needed by the liver to metabolise fats successfully. As its name implies, methionine contains a methyl group and this is particularly important in detoxification reactions as it can be donated to other compounds, including toxins, thereby reducing their toxicity. It is also used to synthesise cysteine and taurine, and, combined with another amino acid lysine, it can be made into carnitine. It is an excellent lipotrophic agent. For instance it is needed for the production of compounds needed for healthy joints. So it benefits the liver in many ways, and is known to help resolve problems involving faulty fat metabolism, fatty livers and high blood levels of cholesterol or triglycerides.

SAM is used by the liver to metabolise excess amounts of oestrogen and so is useful in the treatment of many types of PMS, and in Gilbert's syndrome, a condition in which the blood level of bilirubin is raised. This affects up to 5 per cent of the population, though often without obvious symptoms other than a general malaise.

Taurine

Taurine plays a different role from that of methionine and cysteine. It is not a component of most protein foods, instead it is made in the liver with the help of cysteine and methionine. It then combines with cholesterol derivatives and is made into the bile acids and salts that are essential components of bile. Thus if there is a deficiency of these two amino acids, or if the conversion does not occur correctly and you have insufficient taurine, and if your production of bile seems faulty, you could benefit from a supplement of taurine itself.

Taurine is also important in detoxification processes, not least of them the proper elimination of compounds that can be transported out of the body, with the bile. High cholesterol levels, for instance, can be reduced when the intake of taurine is increased. Taurine also combines with a number of different toxins such as drugs, or compounds the liver has processed, and aids in their elimination. People with food intolerances and poor liver function commonly respond to taurine supplementation.

Glutamine

Glutamine is a derivative of the amino acid glutamic acid and can pick up the ammonia produced during amino acid breakdown and transport it to the kidneys for elimination. Another benefit, important if you are trying to lose weight, is that glutamine can help to reduce cravings for substances such as sugar and alcohol. This means it can also help you to improve your diet and decrease the load of toxins you might otherwise deliver to the liver.

Glutathione

Glutathione contains three amino acids, one of them being cysteine, and it improves the capacity of your liver to detoxify environmental pollutants, drugs and other chemicals. It can convert fat-soluble toxins into water-soluble toxins for elimination via the urine, thus decreasing the work of your liver and the need for their elimination via the gall bladder and bile duct and avoiding the possibility of their reabsorption from the digestive tract. Glutamine helps boost immune function, is a powerful antioxidant and helps to slow down the ageing process.

Carnitine

Carnitine, as its name implies, is found mainly in animals. It is important for the normal transport of fats through the blood and, more particularly, into the mitochondria of cells, where they are converted into energy.

Without carnitine you could have a high level of fat circulating in your blood, which would be bad for your heart, but none going into the cells. As a result you would be tired but gaining weight, probably saying, 'Even when I do eat I don't seem to get any more energy.' The risk of a carnitine deficiency is high among vegetarians and vegans, who may benefit from a supplement. It can also be made in the body, but for this methionine is essential, as is vitamin C.

Carnitine has been shown to be particularly effective in the treatment of alcohol-induced fatty liver, a condition which often shows no symptoms until very far advanced, and if you drink *any* alcohol you should bear this in mind.

What to Drink

Water

Drink approximately four pints or nearly two litres of purified water daily. You can buy the water or you can purify your own. If you do the latter you should use distillation or the reverse osmosis method, not filtering. This is because filters do not remove as many different substances. Distillation requires electricity. The major difference between reverse osmosis and filtering is that as soon as you use a filter it begins to collect the filtered substances and become 'dirty'. In the reverse osmosis method the unwanted substances are constantly removed, with the waste water, while pure water is collected from a separate outlet. Any good supplier of water purifiers should be able to help you with more information about this.

If you don't have your own purified water to hand, buy mineral water. Choose still rather than sparkling mineral water, as the latter contains added phosphates that can have an adverse effect on your calcium levels. The swallowed gases may also cause digestive problems.

Drinking this amount of water confers several benefits. It will help to flush out the toxins, it benefits your kidneys and liver and it will help to reduce your appetite – try drinking two or three glasses of water when you are hungry. It is also essential for normal bowel movements, as you need the fluid to combine with the fibre in your diet. A further benefit concerns your brain. It is thought that insufficient fluid intake can contribute to loss of memory and to senility.

Fluids that Favour your Liver

The Cleansing Cocktail on page 77 contains aloe vera juice for healing, grapefruit seed extract that is anti viral and anti bacterial, and propolis tincture that is antifungal. You will be drinking this during Weeks 1 and 2. If you have candidiasis, continue to drink it but omit the grapefruit seed extract.

By making Lemon Water (see page 77) you can add a pleasant flavour preferable to drinking plain water. The white pith of the lemon also contains limonen, which is good for your gall bladder.

Dandelion coffee is the most readily available and easy to prepare drink, served hot or cold, that is extremely beneficial to your liver and gall bladder in several aspects of this Liver Detox Plan. Get into the habit of having this as your main hot drink .

Green tea contains catechin, a bioflavonoid which aids the liver, is a strong antioxidant and assists the process of detoxification. It is helpful in dealing with allergies and gives a boost to the immune system. Buy the decaffeinated variety and drink it occasionally.

Many herbal teas provide health benefits as well as interesting flavours and are very much better for you than regular coffee or tea

Fruit juices have their place, but they are high in sugar and low in fibre, so drink them in moderation. Eating the whole fruit is better from a nutritional point of view. Ideally you should juice the fruit yourself as there are very few commercial ones that don't have some additives, or lose some nutrients in the processing. Beware of fruit juices made from concentrates, as these can have a number of different chemicals and preservatives in the concentrate which do not need to be listed or acknowledged on the label of the reconstituted juice.

Follow your Appetite

Pay attention to the messages you get from your body, but only to a certain extent. Ignore it when it asks for sugar and fat-laden foods and others that have been banned. Eat only when hungry, not when your taste buds are crying out for the latest pleasure. Furthermore, if, part way through a meal, you have had sufficient, then leave the rest. This is not a crime and, if you want, the remainder can be stored for later. At other times, if you are genuinely hungry then do eat, even if it is not yet meal time. Going for too long without food can lead to hypoglycaemia, with its unpleasant symptoms, and when the time does come to eat, you may be so hungry your will-power will buckle and you will eat foods you shouldn't.

If you want to lose weight as well as to detox, don't focus on that thought. When you focus on how much you are eating, how many calories you have had in the day, whether or not you are 'allowed' more food, then food becomes an obsession. Focus instead on your desire to improve your health, to be fit and healthy. Focus on thoughts of the benefits the permitted foods will give you and the fact that you don't want the harm that the toxic or non-nutritious foods will do to you. Fill yourself up with health-giving and cleansing fruit and vegetables and you will have less room for the calorie-dense foods such as sugars and fats. You will then find the weight coming off steadily and without effort.

Allergies

There is one further point about food selection. If you do have food allergies or sensitivities, or if you suspect that you have them, then avoid the offending foods. You should also avoid foods to which you are addicted or for which you have strong cravings. Allergens often affect the brain in a way similar to the opiates and trigger an addictive response. If there are foods which you claim you simply could *not* do without, eliminate them, at least for a while. They may be causing you problems.

Don't Eat When Stressed

The instructions your brain gives to the rest of your body, via the nervous system can be divided into two main groups. The first group, relating to the sympathetic nervous system (SNS), instructs the body to deal with the outside world. It is your 'fight-or-flight' mechanism. This directs all your resources, hormones, blood flow, lymphatic drainage, etc., to your limbs, heart, lungs and eyes and away from your abdomen.

The second group of instructions, relating to the parasympathetic nervous system (PSNS), instructs your body to pay attention to internal housekeeping. When this system is operating your resources are aimed at producing digestive enzymes, bile from the gall bladder, peristaltic action to move the digestive process along, and a generous blood supply to the abdomen for the absorption of food. It also stimulates the production and expulsion of waste material, both as stool and urine.

The two systems cannot both operate at the same time. Nor can you turn on the PSNS. All you can do is affect the SNS. When you are active, mentally, physically or emotionally, the SNS is on and the PSNS is off. When you relax the SNS turns off and the PSNS comes on. This means that if you are stressed, anxious, irritable or rushing around trying to do things, you should not eat, as your SNS will be on and no resources will be directed at the digestive process. You will get indigestion, damage the lining of your digestive tract, fail to absorb the nutrients you need and even, possibly, generate toxins.

Now you know the reason stressed business people get ulcers. Don't emulate them, don't eat when stressed, do relax before and immediately after you eat.

Herbs

There are many herbs that have specific and beneficial effects on the liver. They are discussed below with, where appropriate, useful suggestions as to how to use them. You won't want to take them all, so pick ones that you think suit you. Some are more readily available than others and this may dictate your choice. You may also find, in your local health food shop, some herbal combinations specifically for the liver. This is the reason I have given you a brief picture of so many different herbs. If you find a remedy with several of them in you can be sure your liver will benefit.

Few people like taking medicines so, where possible, incorporate these herbs into your diet. You may, for instance, be able to grow some at home and add the leaves to salads. Dandelion you can buy ready to make into a drink.

Don't be afraid of the herbs we call spices. The only one that is really spicy is chilli, the rest add all the interesting flavours. Most of them have a wonderfully beneficial effect on your digestive system. The seeds of herbs such as aniseed, cardamom, caraway, coriander, cumin, dill and fennel are excellent for the relief of flatulence. If you are prone to indigestion or flatulence, place a small bowl of mixed seeds on the dining room table and chew on them after a meal. The leaves of basil, marjoram, mint and oregano also aid digestion. Ginger helps to reduce flatulence and relax tension in the digestive system and can be added to a variety of dishes. Horseradish aids digestion, helps to relieve wind and flatulence and is a diuretic and thus promotes elimination via the urine.

Table 3: **Herbs that are good for your liver**

Balmony: stimulates the whole digestive system and helps to prevent constipation. It stimulates the flow of bile for fat digestion and helps in the treatment of gallstones or an inflamed gall bladder. It is an excellent liver herb and has been used in the treatment of jaundice.

Barberry: is one of the best liver herbs. It encourages bile flow and is used in the treatment of gallstone or an inflamed gall bladder and of jaundice.

Black root: is useful when the liver is sluggish and there is severe constipation.

Blue flag: helps the liver and helps prevent constipation but it also helps detoxification in general, being used in the treatment of skin problems when they are associated with a sluggish liver. Such herbs are known as blood cleansers.

Bogbean: stimulates the flow of digestive juices and of bile and helps prevent constipation. It is important if the toxicity is associated with fatigue, arthritis or rheumatism, but you would be better with a different herb if you have diarrhoea or colitis.

Boldo: is useful if you have gallstones or an inflamed gall bladder. If it is in a combination remedy it will be helpful, but should not be your first choice if you are picking single herbs to use.

Cat's claw: is not always thought of as a liver herb. However it is an excellent digestive tonic and is effective against unwanted bacteria and other organisms in the digestive tract, thus helping to re-establish the desirable organisms such as lactobacillus acidophilus and bifidobacteria. It also helps the immune system.

Chelidonium: most herbal remedies are best known by the herb's common name, in this case Greater Celandine, whereas the homoeopathic remedy made from the same plant is known by the Latin name. However this plant, even as a herbal preparation, is best known, in regard to its therapeutic action, by its Latin name, *Chelidonium*. You will find it as a large yellow-flowered poppy-like plant, growing along fences and hedges and by the side of the road. It is beneficial if you have an inflamed gall bladder or gallstones and works well in combination with other herbs, such as dandelion and milk thistle.

Dandelion: one of the best known liver herbs, and one that is readily available. It goes by the botanical name of *Taraxacum officinale*, *Taraxacum* comes from *taraxos*, meaning 'disorder', and *akos*, meaning 'remedy', because it is the remedy for so many disorders in different parts of the body, while *officinalis* confirms its place as an important medical herb. It contains many useful compounds beneficial to the liver including choline. Dandelion triggers both the contraction of the gall bladder and the flow of bile into the digestive tract. In this way, it improves gall bladder function and, as a result, digestion. Since the flow of bile stimulates normal peristaltic action of the digestive tract and hence generate proper bowel movements, dandelion will also help to prevent constipation. Furthermore it has been found to reduce the incidence of gallstones; this may result from its overall benefit to cellular metabolism, as well as to its stimulation of the normal flow of bile.

It acts on the liver as well as on the gall bladder. It improves liver congestion and reduces toxicity, jaundice and hepatitis, and has been used successfully in the treatment of congestive jaundice. In addition to these benefits it acts on the kidneys and helps to prevent fluid retention, being a strong diuretic. As a balance to this action it is also a rich source of potassium, thus it can help in cases of high blood pressure.

You can buy it as tea or coffee and as dandelion preparations from most health food shops. These include tinctures and fluid extracts (concentrated extracts in alcohol), tablets, or gelatine capsules containing the powdered herb. Many of these contain both the leaves and the roots. You will also find dandelion in many preparations designed to treat the liver where it is combined with other herbs and nutrients.

Fringetree: is a herb of general benefit to the liver and gall bladder and helps to relieve any associated constipation.

Fumitory: has a remarkable effect on the liver and gall bladder. It stimulates the flow of bile when this is needed, but if there is already excessive flow, then it reduces this. Finally, if the bile flow is normal then
the herb has no effect. It can be helpful if migraines are associated
with liver problems or when there are problems with detoxification.

Golden seal: has multiple uses. It aids digestion, improves the health of
the mucous membranes lining the stomach and intestinal tract and is
a gentle laxative. This means you can use it if you also have colitis or
a stomach or duodenal ulcer. In addition to toning and benefiting the
liver it will help if your problems include eczema, catarrh, excessive
menstruation and if you have a poor appetite.

Marshmallow root: is rich in mucilaginous compounds which help to
protect and heal any damage to the mucous membranes of the
intestines (damage is likely if you have been subjecting yourself to a
diet high in harmful substances and processed foods).

Milk thistle: also known as silymarin, after one of its constituent
bioflavonoids, or as a corruption of its botanical name, *Silybum mari-
anum*, is a very important liver herb. Like everything else, herbs
have their fashions. Milk thistle used to be used extensively for
liver problems, then it went largely ignored. More recently its active
ingredients have been determined, including silymarin, and as a
result its tremendous benefit to the liver has been recalled and it is
now in common use again.

It stimulates protein synthesis and reduces fatty degeneration of
the liver, particularly when caused by alcohol, and has produced
good results in the treatment of hepatitis and cirrhosis.

It is part of the detoxification process, it protects the liver from
toxins and from free radicals and oxidation and from damage to
the P450 detoxification enzyme system, stimulates the liver's repair
and regeneration and aids its function. It helps maintain glutathione
peroxidase levels and as such is important in antioxidant reactions
and in the fight against free radicals. It is a good herb to use if you
also have skin problems, including psoriasis.

As well as stimulating the flow of bile, milk thistle stimulates the
flow of breast milk (when appropriate) and can safely be used if you
are pregnant or breastfeeding. It can be obtained in tablet or tincture
form and is a common component of many liver remedies, usually
referred to as either 'milk thistle' or 'silymarin'. The seeds can be
made into a tea.

Schizandra: is an extremely valuable herb and gives a deep boost to
the immune system (more so than Echinacea, which is in common
usage) and protects the liver from toxins.

Turmeric: is best known as the spice in Indian food that gives it a yellow colour but it also has healing properties. The yellow pigment, derived from the root, stimulates gall bladder action and the flow of bile. The whole plant is used in the treatment of jaundice and liver disease and may aid the flow of stomach acid.

Vervain: protects the liver and can be used in jaundice and for inflammation of the gall bladder. Choose it if you are also stressed, tense and anxious, or depressed.

Wahoo: is another very important liver herb. It is useful for a congestive liver, increasing the flow of bile and being used to treat the gall bladder problems and gallstones. For the liver it has been used in the treatment of jaundice, and to stimulate normal liver function. This is another herb to use if you have associated skin problems.

Wild yam: stimulates the gall bladder and is helpful in conditions in the digestive tract such as colic and diverticulitis. It is the herb of choice if you also have period problems and pain, or rheumatic problems.

Yellow dock: is a blood cleanser and also works on the liver, helping to prevent congestion and stimulate the flow of bile and useful if you are constipated. Use it if there are associated skin conditions.

It is difficult to generalise and say which of these herbs are the best to use, but if you have other problems pick the liver herb that covers them as well. For instance if you have migraines you might pick fumitory but if you have period pains you might prefer to use wild yam. Otherwise the first choice of herbs for a liver and gall bladder detox programme should probably come from barberry, chelidonium, dandelion, milk thistle, schizandra and wahoo. You will also have to find out what is readily available to you. You may find several different brand-name products that already have a combination of liver herbs in them. Using the above information you should be able to choose the one you think will be best for you.

Tissue Salts

There are 12 tissue salts, all of them mineral combinations found in the body, all used in homoepathic dilutions and all being used to treat different clusters of symptoms, some of which involve the liver and detox processes. They are also generally available in many health food stores, as are small booklets about them if you would like to know more. They are included here for people who like to work with them.

Table 4: **Tissue salts that are good for your liver**

Nat sulph 6x: is the major tissue salt for the liver itself and stimulates the flow of bile. It also improves the liver's ability to remove toxins from the blood and relieves nausea.

Silicea 6x: is an excellent blood cleanser and detoxifier, helping to eliminate deep-seated waste material. It helps bring boils and pimples to a head and release the toxins.

Supplements

Some people say they should be able to get all the nutrients they need from their food. This is true, you *should*, but that does not necessarily mean that you *do*. Manufactured and processed foods are greatly depleted in nutrients compared to foods that grow naturally, are picked ripe and eaten fresh and unprocessed. Furthermore, if you need a detoxification programme you need even greater amounts of many nutrients than you would need simply to maintain good health. Taking the appropriate supplements is the best way to get the additional amounts, while at the same time altering your diet to ensure it provides the greatest amount of nutrients of which it is capable.

The Liver Detox Plan *will* work for you without supplements. However it will work very much *better* if you do follow the suggested supplement programme. You can either take supplements solely while on the detox programme, or you can help to secure maximum benefit long term by continuing with at least some of them on the maintenance programme. The appropriate supplements are given with each section of the detox programme. The following gives you one or two selected comments on the benefits to the liver of some of the specific nutrients. This is not a complete list of what each nutrient does, to list all their benefits would take a book in itself.

Before investing in supplements it is wise to get some advice. They can be a considerable outlay and you want to get the best value you can for your money. To try to assess which you will purchase keep in mind that even before you add in the cost of the nutrients themselves the manufacturing company has basic costs. These include all the overheads, the staff, rent, equipment and so forth; there is the basic cost of physically making a tablet, the cost of making or buying the container and printing and pasting the label. There are also the costs of packing the products and delivering them to the shop and the administration costs involved in running the accounts. These costs are the same whether you buy a product containing small amounts of a few ingredients or a product containing large amounts of lots of ingredients. In other words the cost of the ingredients is only a small part of the total cost.

Why is this worth mentioning? It means that so called 'cheap' products are often a very expensive way of getting the nutrients you want. For instance, you can find on the shelves many low-priced B complexes, containing around 2–5 mg of most of the B vitamins and selling for, perhaps half the price of a B complex containing 50–100 mg of the B vitamins. In other words you could be getting 20 times as much and paying only twice the price. Furthermore it is common to find that the cheap supplements have only a few ingredients, perhaps not even all of the B vitamins, whereas the stronger products tend to have many other associated nutrients as well, such as choline and inositol, other cofactors, synergistic herbs and so forth. It is similar with vitamin C.

It is disheartening to spend money on low-dose or inadequate products, only to find you are not getting the results you had hoped for. So, invest in the best quality products you can afford. Some health food shops have naturopaths on staff, or people with at least some nutritional training – ask their advice as to the best quality brands. You will probably get the best advice from health food shops that specialise in supplements, rather than in ones that specialise in foods. If you want to be very thorough, you could visit a nutritionist or naturopath. Tell them beforehand why you are coming, that you would like advice on particular brands or types of products and make sure they feel confident giving this. If you don't want a full treatment, let them know this in advance.

(It would be helpful for you to refer to Section 2, where we discussed the activation and conjugation steps in the detoxification process, and the nutrients needed for each of them.)

Table 5: **Nutrients that are good for your liver**

Bioflavonoids and OPCs: important antioxidants, needed for activation.

Carnitine: for fat transport into cells.

Carotenoids: beta-carotene and the other carotenoids, the precursors to vitamin A, are important antioxidants and thus assist the detoxification programme, and are needed for the activation step. They are known to help prevent cancer, and reduce the damage of carcinogens.

Coenzyme Q10: improves the oxygen supply to the liver, increases its energy and is protective.

Copper: an important coenzyme for an enzyme called SOD in antioxidant reactions and essential for energy production in all cells.

Cysteine: for the liver, formation of taurine, conjugation.

Glutamine: ammonia metabolism, reduces sugar and alcohol cravings.

Glutathione: is an important antioxidant and aids liver detoxification.

Glycine: needed for the conjugation stage.

Iron: needed for activation as well as for energy production in all cells, including those of the liver.

Lecithin, choline, inositol and serine: are closely related, with most lecithin preparations containing either choline, inositol or serine. They are vital to liver function and needed by the liver for the metabolism of all fats, including both triglycerides and cholesterol. Lecithin contains linoleic and linolenic acids, the essential fatty acids needed for all cell walls including those of the liver. It can be eaten as granules, which should be fresh and stored in an airtight container in a cool place, or taken as a supplement in an oil-filled capsule. Phosphatidyl choline is even more beneficial than lecithin, but it is also a lot more expensive.

Magnesium: needed for both activation and conjugation.

Manganese: an important coenzyme for an enzyme called SOD, involved in antioxidant reactions.

Methionine: a methyl donor, used in the formation of taurine, carnitine and choline, needed for conjugation

Molybdenum: needed for activation.

N-acetyl cysteine, or NAC: is the active form of cysteine, an important sulphur-containing amino acid that is part of glutathione. It helps prevent against toxin-induced cell death and protects the liver from damage. Although NAC is generally more expensive than cysteine it is considerably more beneficial and is usually the most cost-effective way of taking cysteine.

N-acetyl glucosamine, NAG: is the active form of glucosamine sulphate. It helps protect the lining, and encourages the growth of good bacteria in your digestive tract and improves immune function. It is commonly thought of as a remedy for connective tissue disorders such as painful necks and backs, and arthritis. However it is also active in the liver, helping to prevent liver peroxidation and in one study, helped to reduce the size of a tumour in the liver.

Selenium: is probably the most important mineral antioxidant and is essential for the liver's management of free radicals. It is needed for both the activation and conjugation steps.

Taurine: needed for the synthesis of bile salts; for glycine for activation.

Vitamin A: needed for the activation step of detox.

Vitamin B complex: all the B vitamins are needed by the liver, in fact it even stores them, to a small extent, as is evident from the fact that liver in the diet is an excellent source of B vitamins. Additional amounts of B1 will help to reduce sugar cravings, B3 will help to normalise your cholesterol level if it is high. B2, B3 and B6 are needed for the activation step of detox and B6, B9 and B12 for the conjugation step. A lack of these vitamins will lead to fatigue, mental and emotional problems, a variety of skin problems and more.

Vitamin C: an important water-based antioxidant and needed for activation. It is needed for the conversion of cholesterol into bile and the conversion of LDLs to HDLs, for your liver and for detoxification, it also helps to keep blood cholesterol in solution and may help to mobilise it from atheromas. It is needed for the immune system and cleansing reactions.

Vitamin E: an important fat-soluble antioxidant, thus protecting fatty tissues. Needed for activation.

Zinc: needed for activation. An excess of vitamin A can cause problems for the liver, but an accumulation of it can be prevented if sufficient zinc is available for the production of its transport protein. A co-enzyme for the SOD enzyme.

Digestive Enzymes

Digestive enzymes occur in the stomach, the duodenum and the small intestine. They are vitally important for the breakdown of fats, proteins and carbohydrates, and their production can decrease not only with age but with poor health. If you experience a feeling of heaviness or fullness after meals, you may be lacking in hydrochloric acid, digestive enzymes, or both.

Most people produce diminishing amounts of stomach acid as they get older but fail to recognise this. They may even think they have too much acid, since they may experience feelings of acidity or burning. Taking alkalis (antacids) to neutralise the acid further aggravates the problems. The most likely explanation for any burning is that the protective lining of the stomach or oesophagus has been damaged, and the acid that *should* be there is now penetrating through the protective lining to the lower layers that react to the acid. If this applies to you, the aloe vera juice and slippery elm powder you will be taking on the Liver Detox Plan will help to correct this situation.

Hydrochloric acid and enzyme production can be increased by a proper diet and an adequate supply of nutrients such as the B group of vitamins and several trace minerals. In addition you may need to take supplements of enzymes and acid initially. By the end of the programme you may find that your output has increased and you recognise that you are digesting foods much more easily, in which case you can reduce or stop taking these supplements – unless of course the indigestion then returns or you start to slip back into your old ways.

You can purchase the acid and enzymes either separately or in combination. They should be taken *with the end of meals*. This way there is maximum stimulation by the smell, taste and presence of food and the flow of saliva, for the production of your own stomach acid and digestive enzymes and these can work on the first part of the meal. Then when the supplements come along at the end of the meal, when the flow of your own acid is decreasing, they can do their job. (If the meal is only light, consisting of fruit, or a simple salad without protein, you will probably not need them.)

Exercise

Most people live a life that is far too sedentary. Whatever you are doing now, compare it to the way you would have lived in prehistoric times, when there was no transport but your own legs and when you were physically active all day long. Few people are this active today. So if you want to be healthier than you are now, be more energetic than you are now.

The best exercise is the exercise that is built into your daily routine, that occurs throughout the day and that has you breathing more heavily than usually but not to the point where you have to stop to get your breath back. Jog, don't sprint. Aerobic exercise is the best. Run up stairs, walk to the shops. Do stretching exercises in between all your other activities. If you give it some thought there will be many different ways you can build exercise into your life.

Apart from being good for your general health, exercise stimulates the flow of blood down all the capillaries, carrying nutrients to and rubbish from the furthest reaches of your body. It also stimulates your lymphatic system and this helps enormously in mobilising and eliminating toxins.

As a minimum, do 20 minutes of steady exercise twice a day, sufficient to get you puffing slightly.

The Healthy Weight Loss and Liver Cleansing Diet

The Liver Detox Plan is a simple programme that combines delicious recipes with the best of health. It will take you through a detox regime that is gentle and safe. By the end of it you will feel like a new person – though early results will start to come sooner than that.

The Liver Detox Plan is very flexible and there are several ways you can use it. The Short Version consists of Weeks 1, 3 and 5 followed by The Future; The Long Version consists of Getting Started, Weeks 1–6, followed by The Future.

These are some of the options:

Total Commitment

If you want to be as healthy as you can possibly be, as fast as you possibly can and with a good long-term outcome:

1. Follow The Long Version from the Introduction through weeks 1 to 6 to The Future maintenance programme.
2. Stick precisely to the dietary instructions given.
3. Take supplements of all the nutrients indicated.
4. Take a herbal supplement including several of the herbs indicated, with particular emphasis on barberry, chelidonium, dandelion, milk thistle, schizandra and wahoo.
5. Avoid all toxins, as far as you possibly can.
6. Exercise regularly for at least 20 minutes twice a day.
7. After Week 6 follow the guidelines outlined in The Future with regard to both diet and supplements *and stick to them* on a long-term basis.

Congratulations, top marks and good health!

A Quick Fix as Fast as You Can

If you want some results, and fast, but know you won't stick to a long programme, and if you don't feel you have the commitment to make too many major long-term changes but are willing to make some:

1. Follow Weeks 1, 3 and 5, and do at least one week of The Future.
2. Take as many supplements and herbs as you are willing to take.
3. Change your lifestyle for at least the three weeks you are on The Short Version of the Liver Detox Plan.
4. At the end, decide which beneficial changes you could make and maintain long-term and put them into operation.

An acceptable compromise – well done, enjoy the improvements you've made!

A Few Interruptions

You may be serious about wanting to follow the Liver Detox Plan but find that you have social engagements or times when you feel you just cannot stick to it. Don't worry (that won't achieve anything anyway). Stick to it as much as you can and make sure you are not using the distractions as excuses. Whenever you can, get back onto the programme and continue. If you feel you have broken it too seriously, simply go back to the start and begin again. You will eventually accomplish it. Then do all you can to stick to The Future maintenance programme as much as possible. Occasionally you might want to start again and repeat the process for a spring clean.

1. Don't beat yourself up or give yourself a hard time.
2. Use either The Short Version or The Long, depending on your temperament.
3. Follow the programme as much as you possibly can. You may cheat a little each day, but try to do so as little as possible. If you have social distractions, relax, eat as well as you can, then get back onto the programme.
4. Think of some beneficial changes you *would* be willing to make and keep.
5. Acknowledge your achievements.

No Sticking Power

This approach is characterised more by wishing than by determination, but it's better than nothing!

1. Follow Weeks 1, 3, 5 and The Future (Short Version), more or less.
2. Invest in a multivitamin and mineral supplement and a herbal remedy for the liver. (Buying any more supplements than this and then not taking them can put you off.)
3. Stick to the programme as well as you can, backtrack as often as necessary.
4. Acknowledge your achievements.

Anyone can stick to the Liver Detox Plan for a short while, so give it your best shot. Every small improvement you make will improve your health at least a tiny amount, even if it is not obvious at the time.

Self-delusion

As with all programmes, some people will claim they have started on it, stuck to it, yet not gained any benefit, when in fact they have made relatively few changes and have cheated outrageously (and often unconsciously). I have had many patients who have insisted to me that they have made significant changes in their diet but their health hasn't changed, or who insist they have cut their food intake in half and not lost weight. I now get them to write down every single thing they eat and drink on a chart and bring it in for me to see. The results generally surprise both of us.

I recall one patient who did this and said, as the paper lay between us, 'See, I only eat one meal a day and replace the other two meals with a weight-loss drink, I've eaten nothing else.' Yet looking down I could see the sausage rolls at morning tea time, cakes in the afternoon and late-night chocolate biscuits. Finally she laughed at herself and said, 'You know, it really is amazing, I truly did think I had stuck with what you had said,' and after that she did. It is all too easy to 'forget' the things you want to.

In one sense there is no real problem with this. You are, after all, entitled to live your life the way you want, no one can force you to be healthier, and of course it is you who will bear (most of) the consequences later if and when your health deteriorates. The problem is that if you truly do persuade yourself that you *did* stick to the programme and that *it*, not *you*, didn't work, you are then blaming the Liver Detox Plan inappropriately, marginalising it and losing it as a possible option for The Future if or when you do decide that you do want a healthy programme to follow and are willing to stick to one.

Emergency Treatment for a Few Heavy Nights

Most people do it. You have a heavy night out, come home, and just know you ate and drank too much and you're in for a helluva hangover in the morning. It seemed a good idea at the time, but now. . .

Try this treatment:

1. If you're sufficiently *compos mentis* when you get home:
    i) Drink one glass of Cleansing Cocktail (see p77), one strong mug of dandelion coffee and as much Lemon Water as you can. Drink at least a pint of liquid, more than that if possible since much of the hangover effect is due to dehydration.

   ii) Take a strong vitamin B complex, containing up to 100 mg of the major B vitamins, one general multivitamin and mineral supplement and 1,000 mg vitamin C.

   iii) Take a day's supply of your chosen probiotics (acidophilus and bifidus).

2. Next morning repeat that treatment and follow the instructions for Week 1.

If it was one night's transgression, go back to the point you had reached on the Liver Detox Plan. If you have had several nights of overeating and over drinking then stick with the instructions for Week 1 for a whole week.

The Liver Detox Plan as described below is The Long Version. It is written as if you were going to start at Week 1 and continue to Week 6 and then follow The Future. It is written for the committed. If you have chosen to follow The Short Version, modify it accordingly.

Getting Started

You are about to make some major changes to your lifestyle. Many of your favourite foods and recipes may have to go. But many exciting and delicious new flavours are going to come in. You will also find that you quickly feel more alive, more alert, 'cleaner' and more supple. You will lose many of your aches and pains, and be able to shed any unwanted body weight with greater ease than ever before. Your looks will improve and your energy will increase. You will still be able to entertain, and though the nature of the food you provide may be different the pleasure of your guests will still be as great. I can say all this with confidence after working with people using this approach for nearly 30 years – and as a result of following the same programme myself.

   Follow the guidelines given below as fully as you can, given your own individual circumstances. If you follow them totally you will achieve the most benefit, but if you can't do everything, don't worry, do the best you can. For instance, organically produced food is the best, but if you simply cannot afford it, or cannot always find what you want, then at least make the changes you can make.

   Keep in mind that it is important to make the changes you can *sustain*. This programme isn't something you do once and then revert to your old ways. This is the beginning of the rest of your life. That is why there is the basic detox programme and then a set of suggestions for the maintenance programme that will follow. Sadly, I have seen a number of patients follow the programme and feel wonderful, only to revert later to their old ways and wonder why they are beginning to get some of their old problems back.

However, if you do have the occasional blow-out, don't despair. It will indeed slow down the end result, you may even find that the symptoms, the hangover, or the I-ate-too-much-of-the-wrong-food syndrome, feels worse, partly because the contrast is greater, but your liver will be getting stronger and your body will be able to cope. It may just take you a few days to catch up with where you were. Do *not* use this as an excuse to stop! Simply repeat the week you are on and then continue.

Throughout the programme I aim to encourage you all I can. After all, if you are going to do this programme it is worth doing it properly. To begin with, it's worth setting a firm foundation, so some initial planning is appropriate.

It is difficult to stick to a good diet if there are bad and tempting foods in the house, so start in the kitchen. If you live on your own this is simple. If you live with a partner you will want them to be as healthy as you. If you have children, it will be even more important to enlist their involvement – you won't want them to grow up with the bad habits you had, or to be heading for an unhealthy future. If you live with other people, try to enlist their support. If they won't support you perhaps they will at least agree to get rid of the temptations. If you have friends who are determined to remain unhealthy, give the offending foods to them, if not, throw the offending foods out. If that disturbs your idea of waste, eat them up this week and get ready to start next week.

Start with the dry food cupboards. Get rid of all the processed foods, those bearing little resemblance to the way the original ingredients grew or were reared, and laden with toxins. You don't need those packets of cereals made from refined grains and made tempting by the addition of sugar. Replace them with a packet of porridge oats, unsweetened muesli from your local health food store or a cereal made from 100 per cent whole wheat or brown rice. You don't need white pasta and white rice – buy the wholemeal or wholegrain varieties. You don't need highly processed tomato sauces, you will be making your own with fresh tomatoes. You don't need tins of soup, laden with fats, refined starch and a host of additives, you can make a delicious soup on your own, any time you want. Cakes, biscuits, desserts, all these should go, so should all those tempting snacks, crisps and roasted nuts laden with fats and trans fatty acids. Give them all away, or have a party. Personally, I don't think your friends should eat them either, but, unless they're going to join you on this programme they probably will do so anyway so they might as well enjoy your hospitality. Next time the fare you provide will be very different – and no less delicious for all that.

If you ever are tempted by your old foods, don't say to yourself, 'I'd love that, but I mustn't,' for your subconscious will simply try to please you by tempting you into succumbing to temptation. Say instead, 'Yuk, I don't want what *that* would do to me.' You are then focusing on the *benefits* of the changes rather than on what you are, or may be, missing.

Move on to the refrigerator and freezer. Fattening, fat-laden and sugar-rich ice-creams and desserts should go, as should any frozen meals there that don't comply with the suggestions already made. Eat them up, give them away or have a dinner party.

I recall one patient's dramatic start to this programme. An affair had ended abruptly and she was devastated, heartbroken and lonely, with time on her hands. She had come to see me for support in this, but she was also tired and run down, so we discussed the Liver Detox Plan as well. Feeling she had had sufficient upheaval in her life I suggested a gentle start. However when she came back two weeks later she was already a changed person. Her face glowed and she looked and sounded more positive. She had decided to make a clean sweep and had taken on the project as a way of taking her mind off her lost lover. Not only had she given up cigarettes, alcohol, coffee, chocolates and sweets, but she had *totally* emptied her kitchen, cleaned and defrosted the fridge, cleaned the cupboards, reorganised the shelves, restocked them only with items from the shopping list below, and started on the programme 100 per cent. She'd stuck to it and had started to walk to work each day, explaining ,'I felt so good in myself, I simply had to use up the energy.'

Go at your own speed, but keep in mind that for everything you feel you are giving up there are twice as many pleasures, benefits and rewards to be had, both in the near and distant future.

So, on to the next step and this is to make a shopping list. Find a source of organically grown foods, not only fruit and vegetables but meats and other produce as well. There may be one in your area, alternatively there are many of them throughout the country that will deliver. Certainly organically grown produce is often more expensive than the commercially grown variety, but then porridge oats are cheaper, per calorie and per nutrient, than the processed cereals. Basic foods cost less than labour intense processed varieties and you will find many other savings when you buy the foods recommended here rather than many of the less-than-nutritious purchases you have been making. In addition, ill health is expensive, both in money and in quality of life.

As well as stocking up on fresh fruit, vegetables and fresh herbs and finding a good source of fresh fish, you will also want to get the supplements that you elect to take. Use the following checklist to prepare your own shopping list. It is frustrating to start on the programme and then find, at a critical time, that you don't have the necessary components or ingredients.

Shopping Checklist

You don't need to buy everything on the lists below. They are intended to prod your memory, so buy what appeals to you. It is frustrating, however, to want a snack or some food that you could eat, depending on the week you're on, and find you have nothing in the house that appeals. So, make sure you have on hand permitted foods that you can enjoy. You will, of course, have at least some of the things in the house already, possibly many of them. Pay attention to what is needed in individual weeks of the programme and don't buy ahead unless you are sure you will not be tempted – and even then, think twice about doing it!

Weeks 1 and 2

Fresh vegetables and fruit: pick the ones you like the best, but refer back to the list of particularly beneficial vegetables and fruit given above. Buy much greater quantities than you have done in the past as these foods are now going to form the major part of your diet. Include generous quantities of onions and garlic for their sulphur compounds (helpful in detoxification), artichokes, fresh ginger, the cabbage family, carrots and beetroot. The fruit should include citrus fruit, apples and pears and only a few bananas. Buy several lemons and limes, as you will be using these instead of vinegar. Avoid potatoes, tomatoes, peppers, aubergines, mushroom, olives, and avocados.

Sprouts: fresh alfalfa sprouts.

Pot herbs: fresh herbs impart more flavour than dried ones. Now that many of your usual flavourings are banned (being chemically based and non-nutritious) you will be looking for other flavours; fresh herbs and spices are an obvious choice.

Dried herbs: to be used only if you cannot get fresh ones.

Spices: peppercorns, cinnamon sticks, whole nutmegs, whole cloves, mace. Buy a generous amount of turmeric as it is so good for your liver.

Salt: you can find balanced mineral salts in health food shops; they contain potassium chloride, magnesium chloride and others, as well as sodium chloride. Use as little as possible.

Oil: olive oil, the best virgin olive oil you can find, cold-pressed linseed oil.

Fish: whole fish, fish fillets or steaks. Buy fresh if you can, alternatively buy frozen fish. If you simply cannot get either then choose tinned salmon, sardines or mackerel (not tuna), preferably in brine, otherwise in plain olive oil. Avoid smoked fish. Include *small* amounts of other sea foods for variety.

Grains: brown rice, brown rice flour, flaked rice, rice cakes.

Others: rice milk, provided it does not contain added ingredients.

Drinks: toasted and ground dandelion root (coffee). Mineral water, preferably still.

Specials: linseeds, ground psyllium hulls, slippery elm powder, aloe vera juice, lecithin granules, digestive enzymes if needed.

Supplements: your chosen nutritional supplements and herbal remedies or tissue salts. Grapefruit seed extract (anti-bacterial and anti-viral), propolis tincture (anti-fungal).

Weeks 3 and 4

Add the following to your shopping list:

Vegetables: potatoes, tomato, peppers, aubergines, avocado pears.

Whole grains: porridge oats, barley, rye, rye biscuits, millet, buckwheat, and flour and pasta made from these.

Poultry: free-range chickens and eggs, organic if possible of course (note that free range does not necessarily mean organically reared). Buy whole birds or segments of poultry, not sausages or other processed meats. Other birds are also acceptable – duck, turkey, goose, etc.

Drinks: green tea and herbal teas, though dandelion coffee and fresh herbs are still better. Oat milk.

Supplements: probiotics such as *Lactobacillus acidophilus, Bifidobacterium bifido.* And anything you can find, and are tempted by, in the health food shop that complies with this week's instructions.

Weeks 5 and 6

Add the following to your shopping list:

Sprouts: fresh sprouts of the various beans and seeds that are now included in the plan, e.g. mung bean sprouts, sunflower seed sprouts, lentil sprouts.

Grains: wheat and corn, wholemeal flour, wholemeal pasta, polenta, corn pasta. Continue to avoid bread.

Legumes: red, yellow and brown lentils, dried beans, including chick peas. Avoid soy and soy products until The Future, as they are more difficult to digest.

Seeds: sunflower seeds, sesame seeds, pumpkin seeds, pine nuts, tahini (sesame seed paste).

Nuts: raw, not roasted or salted – cashews, almonds, brazils, hazelnuts, macadamias, walnuts (not peanuts), nut butters (not peanut butter).

Oils: walnut oil, almond oil, apricot kernel oil, toasted sesame oil (as liked, for flavouring).

Meat: cuts of fresh meat, lamb, pork, beef, etc. Avoid sausages or other processed meats, ham, bacon or other smoked meats.

Others: Anything you can find, and are tempted by, in the health food shop that complies with this week's instructions.

The Future

You can now add the following to your shopping list:

Vegetables: olives, mushrooms, soy bean sprouts.

Legumes: soy beans, tofu, soy milk and other soy products.

Grains: wholemeal bread, commercial muesli and wholemeal cereals (preferably not toasted and with no added sugar).

Dairy products: permitted now, but eat fewer of these than you did in the past. Whole milk (not skimmed), natural (plain) yoghurt, cottage cheese, ricotta cheese, feta, fromage frais.

Meat/fish: you *can* add smoked products such as smoked salmon, to your diet but it is best to avoid the many smoked and processed sausages as they are generally laden with a variety of unwanted chemicals.

Vinegar: apple cider vinegar, wine vinegar, balsamic vinegar and herb vinegar such as tarragon vinegar. Avoid cheap malt vinegar or vinegars based simply on acetic acid.

Salad dressings: because you can now include vinegar you can buy many of the commercial salad dressings and different types of mayonnaise that are available commercially. Select carefully and purchase ones that use olive oil and have few if any chemical additives.

Others: olives, sun-dried tomatoes, pickled vegetables (preferably of the quality generally sold in health food shops).

Drinks: dandelion coffee – the instant variety if you would like this convenience.

Luxuries: in moderation you can now have honey, hard cheeses, dried fruit (fresh is better).

To celebrate: a top-quality bottle of wine, preferably red! But remember, no more than two glasses in any one day, and avoid cheap wines and bulk wines as they contain a lot more unwanted substances than the good ones.

In general it is relatively safe to buy condiments and sauces from health food shops. Your chances of buying foods high in nutrients and low in unwanted and potentially toxic chemicals are certainly much greater in such shops than in other stores, but continue to read the labels carefully.

As far as possible, continue to avoid peanuts, any nuts that have added oil and salt, crisps, refined carbohydrates (white flour, etc.), sugar and foods containing these, most packaged cereals, foods high in fats and processed foods with a list of chemicals on the label.

Allergies and Candidiasis

Food allergies are common, frequently they are also 'masked', that's to say they are sufficiently hidden that you may not recognise their existence even though their effects can be devastating. They can be caused by liver problems, contribute to liver problems or be associated with liver problems. If you know you are sensitive to certain foods or are allergic to them be sure to avoid them, even if they are included in the recipes given for the week you are on. The top twenty most common allergens include wheat, corn, malt, cow's milk, potato, tomato, chocolate, coffee, peanut, soy, bakers yeast and brewers yeast. For this reason these foods have been excluded from the programme until Week 3 (potato and tomato), Week 5 (wheat, corn), The Future (yeasted or fermented products, dairy products, soy) or altogether (coffee, chocolate, peanut).

If you are not sure, but would like to know, you can have allergy testing done. There are several ways of doing this. The best test, at the time of writing, seems to be the ELISE or FACT tests but this field is developing fast. Kineseology may also give some helpful information. Another clue may be to listen to your body. If you get cravings for certain foods you could be allergic to them as allergens often act on the opiate centres in the brain, and, when you go without them you start to experience withdrawals and hence the cravings. Any time a patient tells me they could not go without so-and-so food I tell them they must. The more they protest (the greater their desire for that particular food) the more I insist that they must avoid them. If they do avoid them they will see beneficial results.

Many people have problems with candida albicans, resulting in candidiasis. This problem too, commonly goes unrecognised, yet its effects can also be devastating, physically, mentally and emotionally. For this reason the foods that should be avoided, if candidiasis is your problem, have also been excluded from the Liver Detox Plan until The Future. However if you know that candidiasis is one of your problems you should continue to do without them (See *Overcoming Candida* by Xandria Williams, Element Books).

Summary

If you like to ease gently into things, this is the week to do it. Some people use this time to eat up what is in the cupboard, hating to waste it. Their attitude seems to be that this is the food they have been eating for years, surely one week more or less won't make all that much difference. To an extent, this is true, but make sure you don't lose the impetus to make the changes, and don't use this as an excuse to delay the start and keep following your old ways.

Concentrate on increasing your intake of fruit and vegetables and cutting down on processed foods, fats and sugars, giving your body a taste of what is to come.

When you feel ready, no matter what day it is, move on to Week 1.

Week 1: Serious Detox

This is the start of the serious detox part of the Liver Detox Plan. It is particularly important if you feel you are very toxic, if you have been used to a high consumption of processed foods, fats, alcohol, tea, coffee and chocolate, if you smoke cigarettes and so forth.

Some people like to make a cleansing start by going on a water fast or a juice fast for a few days. This means eating nothing at all and just drinking water or fruit juice. An alternative would be to eat nothing but brown rice and drink pure water. This is an excellent way to start, if you feel like it. However, since few people are prepared to do this I have not made it an integral part of the programme. But, if you do feel like fasting, this is the time to do it.

There is no need to hibernate, but if you can take things easy this week it is helpful. This is not the week, for instance, to be doing a heavy round of social entertaining, going away on business trips, or burning the midnight oil to meet a deadline. Instead, this would be a great week to pamper yourself. Have that massage or facial you have been promising yourself. Go for walks in the country or, if that is not possible, in a park. See a movie you've been wanting to see. If you've been planning to join a gym, do so now and enrol in some of the gentle programmes such as yoga or tai chi. Swim. Curl up with that good book you've been meaning to read. If none of this is possible then just take things as easy as you can and pamper yourself in small ways (but not by eating the wrong foods!) Improving your health marches hand in hand with improving your mood and your enjoyment of life.

Remember to listen to your appetite, eat only when hungry and do have snacks if you seriously need them, but have no more than two courses at any one meal. You will find the foods surprisingly filling and satisfying, although they are generally low in calories. You will also find, unless you work very hard at eating an enormous amount of fruit and vegetables, that you start to lose weight.

If you know you are sensitive to certain foods or are allergic to them, be sure to avoid them, even if they are included in the recipes given for the week you are on.

During this first week your diet consists of **fresh fruit and vegetables, fresh herbs, spices, brown rice, fish and a small amount of virgin olive oil**. If you are allergic to rice use buckwheat instead, however rice is better for most people. The fruit and vegetables will alkalise your body and provide nutrients. Since this is the beginning of your detoxification programme this is the time when it is most important to get organically grown food if you possibly can. The longer the period of time you can stay on food without the added chemicals, the better. If your fruit and vegetables are not organically grown it is important that they are peeled and the peel discarded. Foods in the nightshade family, including potato, tomato, peppers and aubergine, are excluded as many people are allergic to them and because people with any (even unsuspected) tendency to arthritis will benefit from a period without them. Mushrooms are excluded in case you have candidiasis (overt or covert). The fish will ensure you have sufficient protein, the rice will ensure you feel satisfied and the olive oil will give you the essential fatty acids and will stimulate your gall bladder. You will also be taking all the special foods and whatever supplements and herbal remedies you have elected to take.

Prepare your meals using the ingredients listed above. To give you some ideas, choose recipes from the start of each recipes group, as indicated for Week 1. These recipes are intended only as a guide, they are not the only dishes you should eat during this period. With some imagination you will be able to create a variety of interesting meals for yourself.

You will notice the frequent use of vegetables such as garlic, onion, artichoke, beetroot and the cabbage family. This is as much because they are good for your liver as for their taste, though they do contribute to some interesting flavours.

Supplements

The type and quantity of supplements you take will depend on your budget and on your attitude towards taking them. The following suggestions are a conservative general guideline. Ideally, and particularly if your health is not good, if you are a heavy drinker or seriously overweight, or if you recognise that you have absorbed a lot of toxins, you should take all the supplements listed in Table 5 *(p.46)*. If you want further advice on either what or how much to take you could consult a nutritionist or natural therapist as to your own exact needs. You should certainly do this if you have any serious health problem.

If you are taking more than one tablet of any supplement, take them spread throughout the day, i.e. one tablet taken three times a day is more effective than three tablets taken all at once.

It is difficult to make exact recommendations here without (a) knowing more about your individual state of health and needs and (b) specifying brand names, which would not be appropriate.

Herbs: your chosen herbal remedy or remedies.

Multivitamin and mineral supplement: as a minimum take a good-quality supplement twice a day. Take additional supplements depending on your needs.

Lecithin: 1 capsule of approximately 1,000 mg twice a day, you will also be taking at least 1 tablespoon of lecithin granules each day.

Conjugation: if you find the Liver Detox Plan is leading to unwanted detox symptoms, take an additional 1,000 mg of vitamin C, preferably in combination with the bioflavonoids and OPCs, plus additional amounts of cysteine, glucuronic acid, glutathione, glycine, methionine, vitamins B6, B9 (folic acid) and B12, and the minerals magnesium and selenium. You should be able to get these combined within one or two supplements.

Fibre: it is important that you have three loose and easy bowel motions a day. You will be eating a high-fibre diet anyway on this programme, but at least initially you may need additional help, in which case sprinkle linseeds or psyllium hulls on your foods or stir them into water and drink.

On Rising

One or two large glasses of Lemon Water. Try to have five more glasses of this through the day.

Slippery elm powder.

Breakfast

Every day, no matter what, start with a Cleansing Cocktail.

Take your chosen herbs and supplements.

Follow this with one of the fruit dishes such as those listed for Breakfast Dishes, Week 1. Take the time and trouble to present these dishes elegantly. Fruit salad in a plastic bowl is very different from a mixed fruit delight served in a stemmed glass and decorated with mint leaves and an interestingly cut strawberry. It may be the same nutritionally, but the psychological effect is totally different, and psychological benefits are very important.

If you absolutely have no time to prepare anything, have the Cleansing Cocktail followed by one or two pieces of fresh fruit.

Alternatively, if you are not too conservative, have a salad or vegetable dish such as in Salads, Week 1 or Vegetables, Week 1.

If you are constipated, sprinkle some linseeds over your fruit or vegetable dish.

Dandelion coffee, dandelion tea or herbal tea made using fresh herbs.

Mid Morning

Dandelion coffee, roasted. You can add a slice of lemon or mint but do not use milk or honey this week and do not use the instant form of the coffee.

or

Dandelion tea.

If you are hungry, have some fresh fruit or crudités.

Lunch

Lunch and dinner can be interchanged, just make sure that you have one light meal of one course, and one main meal of no more than two courses each day.

Take your chosen herbs, supplements and aloe vera juice.

For your light meal choose a salad or vegetable dish such as those in Salads, Week 1, or Vegetables, Week 1, and add some fish as well, either plain or as a fish dish from Main Dishes, Week 1. It is important that you have sufficient protein as this is needed by your liver for protection.

Digestive supplements if needed.

Dandelion coffee, dandelion tea or herbal tea.

Mid Afternoon

Dandelion coffee, roasted. You can add a slice of lemon or mint but do not use milk or honey this week and do not use the instant form of the coffee.

or

Dandelion tea.

If you are hungry, have some fresh fruit or more crudités.

Dinner

For your main meal of the day, include two courses. Since you have had fruit for breakfast, and possibly been snacking on it through the day, it would be best to have a savoury starter and main course, leaving the desserts for later in the programme. However you can have a main course and a fruit dessert if this suits you better.

Take your chosen supplements, herbs and aloe vera juice.

For your first course choose a recipe from or similar to those in Snacks, Nibbles and Starters, Week 1, and for your main course choose fish or seafood dishes from or similar to those in Main Dishes, Week 1, and vegetables and/or salads from Salads, Week 1 and Vegetables, Week 1.

If you have decided to have a dessert choose from, or one similar to, one of the fruit dishes from, Breakfast Dishes, Week 1, but do not include rice as this will make your dessert too heavy.

Digestive supplements if needed.

Dandelion coffee, dandelion tea or herbal tea.

Supper

One tablespoon of ground psyllium hulls or linseeds. Stir into water or fruit juice and drink quickly.

If you are still hungry late in the evening, choose one of the light fruit dishes (without rice) from Breakfast Dishes, Week 1.

Week 2: Continuing

If possible, you should continue with Week 1's programme for a second week. This is particularly important if you are in serious need of a detoxification programme, if you have been treating yourself badly for many years, if, after reading Section 2, you realise you have a number of problems that could require the Liver Detox Plan or if you have excess weight to lose.

If you have a lot of weight to lose there is no reason why you should not continue with Week 1's meal plan for several weeks. It is an excellent balance of fresh foods, high-quality protein, olive oil and a small amount of grain in the form of rice. It is close to the caveman diet that human beings consumed for hundreds of thousands of years and it is an extremely healthy way to lose weight.

If, on the other hand, you have been treating yourself relatively well, if, after following Week 1 you already feel rejuvenated, and if you have no extra weight to lose, then move on to Week 3. You will also do this if you are impatient and have opted for The Short Version of the Liver Detox Plan.

Week 3: Lighter Detox

A lifetime of errors, even years or months of errors, cannot be fully corrected in one or two weeks. However life is for living and you will want to be expanding your diet. The aim for this week is to continue with a cleansing diet but at the same time to start adding more variety and increasing the number of foods you can eat.

Potatoes, **tomatoes**, **peppers** and **aubergine** can now be included with the vegetables. You may include **avocado pears**, but eat them sparingly as they are high in fat (and calories), even though it is a healthy and relatively unsaturated fat. This will mean that you can probably cook and use many of your usual vegetable recipes. You must still omit pickled vegetables and mushrooms. The new vegetables feature in the dishes given for this week to add variety to your diet rather than because they are particularly good for your liver. Combine these with the other beneficial salads and vegetable dishes from Week 1.

Fish is no longer the only source of protein. **Poultry** and **eggs** are now included. These should be from birds that have been organically reared, as well as being free range. All the cuts should be low in fat, with all visible fat removed.

Legumes are not included yet as they can be difficult to digest and a strain on the liver. Milk and other dairy products are not included as many people are allergic to these; other people find that dairy products lead to the production of excess mucous and catarrh; lactose (milk sugar) can cause diarrhoea in people who have insufficient lactase (enzyme); pasteurised milk can aggravate candidiasis if you are suffering from that problem (and many people are, even without knowing about it).

Grains such as **millet**, **oats**, **barley** and **rye** are included, though wheat and corn are not because many people have hidden food allergies and two of the most common of these are corn and wheat. In case this applies to you, even without you knowing it, it is as well to omit these two grains for a little while longer.

Foods that have been fermented or contain yeasts that could aggravate candidiasis are still excluded, as are sugar and unrefined carbohydrates.

It is important that you keep in mind that this is a detox programme. For this reason you should continue to make fruit and vegetables the main focus of your meals, ideally up to three quarters of your total food intake. The rest should be divided equally between protein foods and grains.

Recipe ideas for this week can come from the Week 3 section of each recipe group as well as the Week 1 section. You can also plan your own meals, based on the ingredients. The recipes given here are intended only as a guide, and are not necessarily the only dishes you should eat during this period. With some imagination you will be able to create a variety of interesting meals for yourself.

More foods are included in your repertoire from now on so you will be able to use many recipes from the books and sources you already have. For this reason fewer recipes are given for this week and Week 5 than for Week 1. When one of your own recipes calls for ingredients that are not permitted this week, consider what substitutions you can make. If they are relatively simple, go ahead. If they would mean major changes, you may find it spoils the dish so save that one for later in the programme when more of the ingredients are permitted. Continue to use fresh instead of dried herbs where possible, particularly if you have candidiasis.

Substitutions

If a recipe calls for milk, use rice or oat milk. If it calls for vinegar, continue to use lemon juice. For white wine, substitute lime juice and for red wine try using a small amount of beetroot juice (very good for your liver). Using barley flour instead of wheat flour is generally satisfactory in most recipes. Dried fruit can generally be replaced by the fresh variety.

Supplements

Herbs: your chosen herbal remedy or remedies.
Multivitamin and mineral supplement: as a minimum take a good-quality supplement twice a day. You can also take additional supplements depending on your needs.

Lecithin: one capsule of approximately 1,000 mg twice a day. Sprinkle one to two tablespoons of the granules on meals.

Probiotics: as directed on the product.

Liver supplement: look for one that contains cysteine (as NAC if possible), methionine, taurine, carnitine, glutamine, glutathione and possibly NAG.

Tissue salts: Nat Sulph 6x and Silicea 6x (optional).

Conjugation: if you find the Liver Detox Plan is leading to unwanted detox symptoms, take 1,000 mg of vitamin C, preferably in combination with the bioflavonoids and OPCs, plus additional amounts of cysteine, glucuronic acid, glutathione, glycine, methionine, vitamins B6, B9 (folic acid) and B12, and the minerals magnesium and selenium. You may be able to get these combined within one or two supplements.

Propolis tincture: if you have candidiasis, take five drops in water three times a day.

Grapefruit seed extract: take as directed on container if you have candidiasis or any type of intestinal infection, otherwise stop taking this.

Fibre: continue to take linseeds and psyllium hulls if needed.

On Rising

One or two large glasses of Lemon Water. Try to have five more glasses of this through the day.

A supplement containing *Lactobacillus acidophilus* and bifido bacteria.

Slippery elm powder.

Linseeds or psyllium hulls if necessary.

Breakfast

If you have candidiasis, continue to take the Cleansing Cocktail.

Take your chosen supplements and herbs.

Choose recipes from or similar to those in Breakfast Dishes, Week 3, as well as Week 1. You can also have any food that has been left over from the day before, such as the remainder of lunch or the evening meal, if that appeals to you and is convenient. Although more satisfying breakfasts, such as eggs on brown rice, are now included, you should continue to include fruit and vegetables in each meal. Vegetables, for instance, can be incorporated into scrambled eggs or omelettes, and fruit can accompany the meal.

Digestive supplements if needed.

Dandelion coffee, dandelion tea or herbal tea.

Mid Morning

Dandelion coffee, roasted. You can add a slice of lemon or mint but do not use milk or honey this week and do not use the instant form of the coffee.

or

Dandelion tea.

If you are hungry, have some fresh fruit or crudités.

Lunch

Take your chosen supplements, herbs and aloe vera juice.

If this is your light meal of the day, choose dishes from or similar to those in Salads, Week 3, as well as Week 1, or Vegetables, Week 3, as well as Week 1. Make sure you have some protein in the form of fish, seafood, eggs or poultry.

Digestive supplements if needed.

Dandelion coffee, dandelion tea or herbal tea.

Mid Afternoon

Dandelion coffee, roasted. You can add a slice of lemon or mint but do not use milk or honey this week and do not use the instant form of the coffee.

or

Dandelion tea.

If you are hungry, have some fresh fruit or crudités.

Dinner

Take your chosen supplements, herbs and aloe vera juice.

Choose a starter from or similar to those in Soups, Week 3 or Week 1, or else Starters, Week 3 or Week 1. Choose your main dish and vegetables or salads from Main Dishes, Week 3, as well as Week 1, and Salads, Week 3, as well as Week 1, and Vegetables, Week 3, as well as Week 1. If you don't have a starter, you can choose a dessert from Desserts, Week 3, or Breakfasts, Week 1.

Digestive supplements if needed.

Dandelion coffee, dandelion tea or herbal tea.

Supper

One tablespoon ground psyllium hulls, stir into water or fruit juice and drink quickly.

If you are still hungry late in the evening, choose one of the light fruit dishes from Breakfasts, Week 1.

Week 4: Continuing

If you can do it you should continue with Week 3's programme for a second week. This is particularly important if you are in serious need of a detoxification programme, if you have been treating yourself badly for many years, if, after reading Section 2, you realise you have a number of problems that could require the Liver Detoxification programme or if you have excess weight to lose.

If you have a lot of weight to lose there is no reason why you should not continue with Week 3's meal plan for several weeks. It is an excellent balance of fresh foods, high-quality protein, oil and complex carbohydrates. It is also sufficiently varied to prevent any charge of monotony.

If, on the other hand, you have been treating yourself relatively well, if, after following Week 3, you already feel rejuvenated, and if you have no extra weight to lose, then move on to Week 5. You will also do this if you have opted for The Short Version of the programme.

Week 5: Final Detox

This is the time to expand your diet further. From now on it will include all the grains so you can now incorporate **wheat** and **corn** into the recipes, but not bread yet, as that contains yeast. You will also be able to eat **red meat**, including **pork**, **lamb** and **beef**. **Legumes** such as **red kidney beans**, **lima beans** or **lentils** can be included, but not soy beans, so can seeds, such as **sunflower seeds** and **sesame seeds**, and **raw nuts**, with the exception of peanuts. You should continue to avoid dairy products, sugar and foods on the list of yeasted or fermented foods.

In spite of the addition of all these relatively 'dry' foods, keep in mind that you are on a Liver Detox Plan. It will be more successful if you keep your diet as simple as possible. You should continue to ensure that three quarters of your diet is fruit and vegetables. In other words, keep to the recipes from Weeks 1 and 3 as far as possible, but use small amounts of the new foods that are included for this week, when you need to. The more successful you are at doing this the more beneficial will be the results. These new foods should be used to provide variety, not to crowd the vegetables and fruit out of your diet.

Use your own recipes, making modifications, if necessary, to remain within the list of permitted ingredients. Recipe ideas for this week can come from the Weeks 1, 3 and 5 sections of each main Recipe Group. These recipes are intended only as a guide, they are certainly not the only dishes you should eat during this period. Choose your foods from those given above and those you were eating in Weeks 1 and 3. Using these foods and some imagination you will be able to create a variety of interesting meals for yourself.

Supplements

Linseeds: if needed.

Herbs: your chosen herbal remedy or remedies.

Multivitamin and mineral supplement: as a minimum take a good-quality supplement twice a day. You can also take additional supplements depending on your needs.

Lecithin: one capsule of approximately 1,000 mg twice a day. Sprinkle one to two tablespoons of the granules on meals.

Liver supplement: look for one that contains cysteine (as NAC if possible), methionine, taurine, carnitine, glutamine, glutathione and possibly NAG.

Conjugation: if you find the Liver Detox Plan is leading to unwanted detox symptoms, take 1,000 mg of vitamin C, preferably in combination with the bioflavonoids and OPCs, plus additional amounts of cysteine, glucuronic acid, glutathione, glycine, methionine, vitamins B6, B9 (folic acid) and B12, and the minerals magnesium and selenium. You may be able to get these combined within one or two supplements.

On Rising

One or two large glasses of Lemon Water. Try to have five more glasses of this through the day.

A supplement containing *Lactobacillus acidophilus* and bifido bacteria.

If you suffer from candidiasis, take the Cleansing Cocktail.

Linseeds or psyllium hulls if necessary.

Breakfast

Take your chosen supplements.

Choose recipes from or similar to those in Breakfast Dishes, Weeks 1, 3 and 5. You can also have any food that has been left over from the day before, such as the remainder of lunch or the evening meal, if that appeals to you and is convenient.

Digestive supplements if needed.

Dandelion coffee, dandelion tea or herbal tea.

Mid Morning

Dandelion coffee, roasted. You can add a slice of lemon or mint but do
not use milk or honey this week and do not use the instant form of
the coffee.

or

Dandelion tea.

If you are hungry, have some fresh fruit or crudités, or a handful of raw
nuts or sunflower seeds. Try Spiced Seeds and Nuts.

Lunch

Take your chosen supplements, herbs and aloe vera juice.

If this is your light meal of the day, choose dishes from, or similar to
those in, Salads or Vegetables for Weeks 1, 3 or 5. Make sure you
have some protein in the form of fish, seafood, eggs, poultry or meat.

Digestive supplements if needed.

Dandelion coffee, dandelion tea or herbal tea.

Mid Afternoon

Dandelion coffee, roasted. You can add a slice of lemon or mint but do
not use milk or honey this week and do not use the instant form of
the coffee.

or

Dandelion tea.

If you are hungry, have some fresh fruit or crudités, or a handful of raw
nuts or sunflower seeds. Try Spiced Seeds and Nuts.

Dinner

Take your chosen supplements, herbs and aloe vera juice.

Choose a starter from, or similar to those in, Starters or Soups for Weeks
1, 3 and 5, a main dish from, or similar to those in, Main Dishes,
Weeks 1, 3 and 5 and vegetables or a side salad such as those in
Vegetables, Weeks 1, 3 and 5 and Salads, Weeks 1, 3 and 5. If you
don't have a starter, you can choose a dessert from or similar to those
in Breakfasts, Week 1 or Desserts Weeks 3 or 5.

Digestive supplements if needed.

Dandelion coffee, dandelion tea or herbal tea.

Supper

One tablespoon ground psyllium hulls, stir into water or fruit juice and
drink quickly.

If you are still hungry late in the evening, choose one of the light fruit
dishes from Breakfast Dishes, Week 1.

Week 6: Continuing

If you can do it you should continue with Week 5's programme for a second week. This is particularly important if you are in serious need of a detoxification programme, if you have been treating yourself badly for many years, if, after reading Section 2, you realise you have a number of problems that could require the Liver Detoxification programme or if you have excess weight to lose. You have come this far, another week before you start The Future could make all the difference.

If you have a lot of weight to lose there is no reason why you should not continue with Week 5's meal plan for several weeks. It is an excellent balance of fresh foods, high-quality protein, oil and complex carbohydrates. It is also sufficiently varied to prevent any charge of monotony.

If, on the other hand, you have been treating yourself relatively well, if, after following Week 5 you already feel rejuvenated, and if you have no extra weight to lose, then move on to The Future. You will also do this if you have opted for The Short Version of the programme.

The Future: Your New Routine

This is the start of your full maintenance programme. The rules are relaxed, but still there. This is no time to go back to your old ways, if you want to be truly healthy you should continue to avoid white flour, white rice, sugar and other refined carbohydrates. Avoid fried and fatty foods. Continue to avoid processed foods and foods with a variety of added chemicals. Ideally you should avoid tinned foods and pre-prepared foods and sauces. In practice you probably won't do this, but if you do eat them, keep them to a minimum. You should still base your diet on fresh foods and prepare them yourself. It is time well spent, and in terms of the health and energy benefits you will receive, you will gain time, not lose it by doing this because you will have more energy for the rest of your life as your health and well-being improve.

Include **soy beans** and **soy products**. If you don't suffer from candidiasis you can now add **dairy products** back into your diet, unless you know you are allergic to them, and the foods made with or containing **yeast** or **fermented products**. While sugar is not a necessary part of the diet, a small amount of **honey** can be used to sweeten the occasional dessert. **Herb teas** and **alcoholic drinks**, including wine are also permitted (in moderation), as are bought **fruit juices**, in addition to those made at home, though the latter are better. You can use the **instant form of dandelion coffee** if you want that convenience. Fruits and vegetables should continue to provide at least 50 per cent of your diet, at all meals.

If you suffer from candidiasis, continue to follow the programme described for Week 5 and take the Cleansing Cocktail (p.77) regularly plus probiotics.

Learn to adapt all your favourite recipes to the above criteria. Ideas for your new routine can come from all those included in the recipe section. Only a few new recipes have been given, since a high proportion of the recipes in your own cookbooks will be available to you now, provided you modify them as appropriate for nutritional benefit.

Substitutions

- wholemeal flour for white flour, wholemeal pasta for pasta made with white flour
- honey (small amount) or fruit juice in recipes instead of sugar
- olive oil, tahini or avocado instead of butter
- natural or Greek (creamier) yoghurt instead of cream
- soft, low-fat cheeses instead of hard, high-fat cheeses
- Tamari instead of commercial soy sauces

This is the ideal plan for your future. In practice you probably won't stick to it absolutely, but do your best. In general, the closer you stick to this, the healthier you are likely to be. When you are eating away from home you may choose to be more flexible, eating, for instance, white pasta or rice in a restaurant. However do not use this 'flexibility' as an excuse to indulge in sugar- and cream-laden desserts. You can still make good choices rather than bad ones (a simple entrée rather than one high in fat or white flour; a side salad or plain vegetables rather than chips and rich creamy sauces; fresh fruit, fruit salad, etc. instead of Black Forest gateau with cream).

Supplements

By now you should be feeling very much better and you can reduce your supplements to maintenance levels. If, however, you notice the difference when you reduce the amount you take, go back on the supplement programme given for Weeks 5 and 6. If you find, after a while on The Future diet and reduced supplement programme, that your diet is deteriorating and that you are tending to go back to your old ways, you should certainly increase your supplements back to the levels of Weeks 5 and 6, whether or not you decide to improve your diet, although that would obviously be a wise thing to do!

Multivitamin and mineral supplement: as a minimum take a good-quality supplement twice a day, possibly some extra antioxidants. You can also take additional supplements depending on your needs

Lecithin: sprinkle one to two tablespoons of the granules on meals.

Vitamin C: 1,000 mg of vitamin C, preferably in combination with the bioflavonoids and OPCs.

On Rising

One or two large glasses of Lemon Water. Try to have five more glasses of this through the day.

Continue to eat linseeds or psyllium hulls for as long as is necessary .

Breakfast

Take your chosen supplements.
Choose from the recipes provided or from permitted foods.
Digestive supplements if needed.
Dandelion coffee, dandelion tea or herbal tea.

Mid Morning

Dandelion coffee (you can now add milk to it if you wish) or dandelion tea.
If you are hungry, have some fresh fruit, crudités, or a handful of raw nuts or seeds.

Lunch

Take your chosen supplements.
Digestive supplements if needed.
Dandelion coffee, dandelion tea or herbal tea.
A light meal of salads or vegetables with some protein. See The Future section of each recipe group.

Mid Afternoon

Dandelion coffee, with milk if you wish.
or
Dandelion tea.
If you are hungry, have some fresh fruit or crudités, raw nuts or seeds or some of the snacks in the recipe sections.

Dinner

Take your chosen supplements.
Digestive supplements if needed.

Dandelion coffee, dandelion tea or herbal tea.

Have two courses, selected from, or similar to any of those given in the appropriate recipe sections, up to and including the recipes for The Future.

Supper

Fresh fruit, plain yoghurt, fruit salad with plain yoghurt and sunflower seeds.

As you get more venturesome you will obviously include other recipes of your own. However you should refer back, from time to time, to the general guidelines given throughout this book as to what constitutes a good or a bad diet and trim your sails accordingly so that you remain healthy and do not need to go back on this programme again.

After the Liver Detox Diet

What do you do if you've been on the programme once but have relaxed too far and need a booster detox, or if you felt better but then find some of your old symptoms returning? You needn't necessarily go back to the start, though that would certainly be of benefit. Here are some specific steps you can take.

You may have followed The Long Version (the serious detox) or The Short Version (if you were in pretty good health and habits to start with), become well established on The Future maintenance diet and then blown it with a night out, rich food, ice cream, chocolate, coffee and alcohol. What do you do? If it's just one day then a day or two on Week 1 meals should help you get back on track. Take the supplements for Week 1 and the additional ones from Week 5. If it has been several days, follow Week 1 for a full week.

Alternatively, you may have stuck with The Future maintenance programme – or at least you think you have. Then you realise that over a period of time you have, step by step, fallen back into some of your old habits and that your health, or at least your general sense of well-being, have begun to suffer as a consequence.

Mild lapses and symptoms might warrant a repeat of Week 1, then a return to The Future and a promise to stay with that. If you slipped up quite a bit but are still following a much better diet than you were before you started on the Liver Detox Plan then it would be a good idea to do The Short Version of the programme. If, on the other hand, you recognise that you have almost, if not fully, reverted to your old ways then some soul searching is needed, and you will have plenty of time to do that during the six weeks of The Long Version followed by The Future.

Foods to Avoid if You Have Candidiasis

If you know or suspect you are suffering from candidiasis or candida-related symptoms, the following yeast-related foods should be totally eliminated from your diet:

- bread, buns, pizzas, yeasted cakes, doughnuts and any other food made with yeast as the rising agent (NB 'yeast-free' breads commonly do contain yeasts and related organisms as the dough is allowed to 'sit' for a while, usually in a bakery in vats open to the yeast-laden air, and 'ferment'. A variety of compounds and gases form in the dough and these provide much of the texture and flavour.)
- fermented grain products such as soda bread (contains soured milk) and pumpernickel bread
- cheese, yoghurt, soured and fermented dairy products
- all alcohol with the possible exception of neat spirits
- vinegar, mayonnaise, salad dressings and any other food containing vinegar (use fresh lemon juice instead)
- pickles, olives
- tomato products such as juice, sauce, purée, paste; also tinned tomatoes (fresh tomatoes can be eaten)
- soy sauce, and most other similar sauces if any of the ingredients have been fermented or include vinegar
- marmite and similar yeast-based spreads
- mushrooms
- smoked foods such as kippers, bacon, ham and smoked cheeses
- malt
- dried fruit
- melons, fresh or dried
- fruit juices, soft drinks
- tinned fruit or commercially preserved fruit
- desiccated coconut and other coconut products
- peanuts, as these are prone to growths of moulds. This includes peanut butter and any other peanut products.
- dried herbs may contain moulds so use fresh ones instead. Spices are generally safe.
- sweet foods to avoid include sugar in any form including table sugar, honey, syrup, rice sugar, maple syrup, fruit juices and cordials
- pasteurised milk should be avoided both because of the sugar it contains (lactose) and because it encourages the growth of candida. Cream is less of a problem, but it is high in fat.

If you do suffer from candidiasis you should continue to follow the guidelines for Week 5 but focus on vegetable dishes rather than fruit and limit your fruit intake to one or two pieces a day.

THE RECIPES

This is not intended as a recipe book. However it is not easy to start on this programme without some help. Most of the recipes you already have will not be applicable at the start and so the following are provided as ideas. Week 1 is the most difficult, so several recipes are given. Week 3 may also be difficult, as you still have to find ways around the absence of bread, sugar or dairy products, so several ideas are provided. As you get to the later weeks and the list of foods you can eat grows you will find you can use more and more recipes in your own recipe books and so fewer examples are given here. Where appropriate, the recipes given in later sections focus on the new foods being brought into the programme for that week.

Above all, keep in mind, that the recipes are general ideas: use them to think of other things you can do with the foods permitted.

Cleansing Recipes

Cleansing Cocktail

Ingredients

50 ml aloe vera juice
*(If the juice you buy is concentrated,
dilute it as indicated and drink
50 ml.)*
5 drops propolis tincture
*(This is antifungal and will act
against any possible moulds,
including candida albicans.)*

2 drops grapefruit seed extract
*(This is anti-bacterial, anti-viral
and also somewhat anti-fungal.)*

Method

Combine these three with water or with fresh fruit juice, made at home. If you have a juice extractor you can choose any fruit you like. If you have a blender, choose a softer fruit, purée it and then add the three ingredients. Citrus juice is, of course, easy to make at home.

You will be drinking this during Weeks 1 and 2. If you have candidiasis you should continue to drink it throughout the programme (and beyond if your problem persists) but omit the grapefruit seed extract after Week 2.

Dandelion

Dandelion, as already discussed, is an excellent liver and gall bladder herb, with additional benefits for the kidneys, and has many benefits in a detox programme. It also makes a pleasant drink hot or cold, and you will find it recommended daily throughout the programme. You can use either the leaves or the root, or of course, a combination of the two, and there are many different ways you can use it. If you have a garden it is worth letting the dandelions grow, either scattered through it as they appear, or by keeping a section of your garden specially allocated to the plant.

Dandelion Salad

Pick the fresh leaves, choosing the younger ones. Wash, tear and add to salads. They are slightly tart and add a pleasing piquancy to mixed leaf salads. They can also be added to other recipes as a chopped herb. Use or add them frequently if you have them available in the garden, even when not specifically mentioned in the salad recipe you are using.

Dandelion Tea

Pick and wash the fresh leaves. Chop finely. Allow a teaspoon per cup, add boiling water and allow to steep for a few minutes. Drink without milk. In The Future you can add a little honey if desired.

Dandelion Coffee

The instant form can be used in The Future; until then, using the roots from your garden involves a little more work. In general they should be dug up between June and September, when they are at both their most bitter and their most beneficial. However you are probably impatient to get started, and it may not be summer right now, so if you have some, dig them up anyway. You already know they are prolific growers and they will soon be replaced in the garden.

Clean them thoroughly, chop them finely, roast them in a warm oven, taking care not to let them burn. Once they are completely dried grind them in a coffee grinder.

Dandelion Coffee, Roasted

Place some of the powdered root in a saucepan with water. You will soon work out the proportions you like. Some patients tell me they like it strong, to get the flavour, other people like it weak, so suit yourself. It is important that you make it the way you like it as you will be drinking it often. Allow it to simmer for up to half an hour, adding more water as necessary. This is a long time, but you don't get a lot of powder for the work you put in and you want to get the most out of it. You can boil it for less time if you prefer and if you are in a hurry. Strain and drink. You can also make a large batch of it and heat it up during the day. Do this if you are away from home during the day.

For many people this may seem like too much hard work, and you will be pleased to know there is an easier alternative. You can buy dandelion coffee in most health food shops, in two forms. One is the roasted and ground root, all you have to do is simmer it for about half an hour, strain and serve. In the other all the work is done for you (see below).

Dandelion Coffee, Instant

This form can be used in The Future. The dandelion root has been roasted and treated so that only the soluble components are presented. It is convenient to use, however it is often blended with lactose (milk sugar). This is fine unless you have a lactose intolerance; if you do, it will cause diarrhoea. Many people with milk allergies are allergic to the proteins in milk, and not the milk sugar, in which case you may be able to drink this quite safely. On the other hand, if you are suffering from candida-related problems and have to cut sugars out of your diet absolutely rigorously, then you may not be able to drink it.

Both types of dandelion coffee have a flavour of their own. They do not taste like coffee. However the flavour, though an acquired taste, is pleasant, the coffee can be drunk at any time of day and it offers the added benefit of what it is doing for your liver.

Fresh Herbal Teas

Dried herbs may contain moulds and so should be avoided if you have candidiasis. However fresh herbs make excellent tea, with a cleaner and sweeter flavour. Many of the herbs you can grow for yourself, either in the garden, if you have one, or in pots. Quantities are not given here as you will soon discover how strong or weak you like them. For the first six weeks you should drink them plain. In The Future you can add a small amount of honey if you wish, though by then you will probably have learnt to enjoy their natural flavours. Most of them, unless other directions are given, can be made simply by pouring boiling water on the leaves and allowing them to steep for 5 to 10 minutes.

A few teas are listed below to give you ideas. Any herbs can be used, depending only on your flavour preferences. None of the teas listed below are as beneficial to the liver as dandelion coffee or tea, but they are cleansing and refreshing and many of them improve digestion. If you can obtain any of the liver herbs fresh, they can be made into teas, with obvious benefits.

Chamomile Tea

Chamomile is easy to grow. It thrives when walked on and can be incorporated into lawns to provide floral interest and a sweet aroma. Chamomile tea is relaxing to the digestion, helps to improve your intestinal flora and can improve sleep.

Dill Tea

Dill is an excellent herb to serve sprinkled over steamed vegetables and can also be used to make a tea that will aid digestion.

Lemongrass Tea

Lemongrass is tall and somewhat tough. Cut it into lengths about 2 cm long, place in a saucepan, add water and simmer for 10 minutes, strain and serve.

Lemon Balm Tea

This also has a pleasantly refreshing flavour of lemon, but the plant is from the mint family and is easy to grow in a pot. The tea is made by infusing the leaves.

Nettle Tea

Nettles, as any country rambler knows, grow wild and can occur in the most unexpected places. Take a pair of rubber gloves with you for protection while collecting. Wash the leaves and add boiling water. You will be pleased to know that once treated in this way they will not sting you any more (hence the safety of nettle soup, too). The leaves are rich in chlorophyll, iron, silica and other minerals and in vitamin C. The flavour of the tea is gentle and it combines well with other herbs such as peppermint. Nettle is of great benefit as a tonic and blood purifier. It stimulates your kidneys and helps in the elimination of toxins.

Peppermint Tea

Peppermint, like most of the mints, is easy to grow. Pick a few leaves when you need them. Peppermint aids digestion and can help if you have an upset stomach. Since it also stimulates the flow of bile and the actions of the liver it is an excellent herb tea to drink during the Liver Detox Plan.

Sage and Thyme

These are two common culinary herbs, easy to grow and frequently used in cooking. Pick a few leaves, pour on boiling water, allow to cool and gargle with them for a sore throat, then swallow. They can also be made into teas in the same way as peppermint. Sage stimulates the flow of bile and helps digestion.

Spice Teas

Seeds such as caraway, cardamom, cumin, dill and fenugreek aid digestion. To make them into a tea, simmer the desired quantity of the seeds in water for 5 to 10 minutes, strain and serve.

Lemon Water

Pure water This can be still or sparkling according to your choice, though still is better as sparkling mineral water contains too much phosphorous.

Lemon Make the effort to get organically grown lemons as you will be using the skins as well as the juice. Cut them into slices and soak them in the water. You will soon work out how much lemon flavour you get and how much you enjoy. If the lemons are not organically grown, do not use the skin; simply squeeze the juice and add to the water.

Variation Use limes instead of lemons.

Linseeds

Linseeds can be swirled into a glass of water and drunk immediately or sprinkled on food just before eating. When added to a fruit salad, for instance, they give you something to chew, but don't allow them to soak in it for so long that the juice starts to thicken (unless, of course, you like that). Alternatively you can put them to soak in fruit juice and, when the mixture has thickened or 'set', eat it like a jelly.

Psyllium Hulls

Psyllium hulls should be bought ground. They can then be consumed like linseeds, either swirled into water and drunk immediately, or mixed with fruit juice and allowed to set into a jelly before eating.

Psyllium Jelly

Ingredients

ground psyllium hulls   freshly squeezed fruit juice

The quantities will depend to a certain extent on the psyllium you buy, and also on whether you like a softer or a thicker jelly.

Method

Stir the ground psyllium hulls into the fruit juice and allow to set.

In addition to providing fibre, this makes a possible 'dessert' or 'something sweet' when you have already had two courses and are looking for something more. It will also help, if you are trying to lose weight, to fill you up using relatively few calories, just those in the fruit juice.

Slippery Elm and Banana

The easiest way to take the slippery elm powder seems to be to mash one teaspoon of pure slippery elm powder (not slippery elm food) into a banana or some other food.

If you prefer you can make it into a paste with water and then drink it.

Breakfast Dishes

Although designed initially as breakfast dishes, many of the breakfast recipes for Week 1 are based on fruit and can also be used as desserts.

Week 1

It is important that you find a pleasant way of taking a tablespoon of lecithin granules each day throughout the whole programme. Experiment by adding them to some of the dishes below and find your favourite way of taking them, even if they are not specifically mentioned in the recipe. They have a slight creamy flavour and often add interest to a dish.

Mixed Berry and Mint Delight

Ingredients

2 oranges, squeezed
5 mint leaves

a selection of berries, in season, such
    as blackberries, raspberries,
    strawberries, blue berries or others

Method

Steep the mint leaves in the orange juice. Wash and prepare the fruit and mix in a bowl. Pour over the orange juice and serve, decorated with a fresh sprig of mint.

Winter Special

Ingredients

1 apple
1 pear
1 banana

1 lemon, juiced
pinch grated nutmeg

Method

If the apple and pear are organically grown, leave the skin on, otherwise remove it. Peel the banana. Chop the fruit, add the lemon juice and toss until the fruit is coated in it. Lightly sprinkle with nutmeg, freshly grated for preference.

Spicy Fruit Salad

Ingredients

1 cup pear or apple juice freshly
made *(If this is not possible, use a
combination of freshly squeezed
orange and lemon juice.)*

1 cinnamon stick
1 clove
pinch of freshly grated nutmeg
fresh fruit of your choice

Method

Put the juice in a saucepan, add the spices, bring to the boil and simmer for 10 minutes, being careful not to let the liquid evaporate away. Allow to cool.

This can be made ahead of time, stored in the fridge, and used as required.

Chop the fresh fruits and mix them together. The dish will look attractive if you are able to combine fruit of different colours.

Add some of the spiced juice, to taste.

Serve in attractive glass dishes.

Wimbledon Blend

Ingredients

1 bunch seedless black-fleshed
grapes, cut in half

1 kiwi fruit, peeled and chopped
1 Granny Smith apple, chopped

Method

Toss the fruit together.

Serve in a bowl lined with purple and green leaves.

Citrus Concerto

Ingredients

1 orange
1 blood orange
1 grapefruit
1 blood grapefruit

1 mandarin
1 tangerine
crisp lettuce leaves
1 lime

Method

Peel all the fruit except the lime and separate into segments.

Lay the lettuce leaves on a platter and arrange the citrus segments over them, alternating the colours to make a pleasing pattern.

Squeeze the lime and drizzle the juice over the fruit.

Fresh Fruit Platter

Ingredients

a variety of fresh fruit in season   crisp lettuce leaves

Method

Prepare the fruit so that it is ready to eat, in bite-sized pieces.
Place a layer of lettuce leaves on a flat platter and arrange the fruit over it.
Decorate with sprigs of fresh parsley.

The remaining recipes in this group include rice and can be eaten if you feel you need a more filling breakfast than one consisting of only fruit or vegetables. Do not use them for desserts (lunch or dinner) unless you have had a *very* light dish for your first course.

Rice Porridge with Apple and Pear

Ingredients

50 g brown rice flour   water or fresh apple or pear juice
1 apple   1 tablespoon lecithin granules
1 pear

Method

Mix the rice flour with sufficient water or juice to make a thick liquid
Place the mixture in the top half of a double boiler and cook over boiling water, stirring occasionally.
Add more liquid if the porridge thickens too much.
When cooked (the time it takes will depend on how fine the flour is), grate the apple and pear and add to the porridge together with the lecithin granules. Stir and cook for another minute.
Serve with more fruit juice.

Fruit and Rice Pudding

Ingredients

170 g brown rice, cooked in water   chopped fresh fruit of your choice
   or fruit juice   1 tablespoon lecithin granules

Method

Combine all ingredients.

Fresh Fruit Rice Muesli

Muesli was originally a fruit dish. This is not quite the full muesli but is a variation suitable for Week 1.

Ingredients per person:

1 tablespoon, approximately, rolled or flaked rice (available from some health food stores)

1 teaspoon lecithin granules

2 pieces of fresh fruit, such as an apple and a pear, or the equivalent *(You could combine a kiwi fruit, a pear and a few grapes, or an apple and a small mango. Choose from the fruit in season and combine them in different ways to suit your taste.)*

fresh fruit juice

Method

Put the rice flakes in a bowl and pour just sufficient hot water over them to soften them. Add the lecithin granules.

Chop the fruit and pile on top of the softened flakes.

Serve with fresh juice if desired.

Variation

If you cannot get rice flakes you could use rice cakes, crumbled into small pieces.

Week 3

Breakfasts for Weeks 3 and 4 can continue to be chosen from those above. However, if you would like something more substantial, choose from one of the following dishes. You can now have eggs and some of the grains so you can have a great variety of breakfasts. The eggs can be boiled, poached, scrambled (use olive oil) or made into omelettes. You cannot have bread yet, but you can now make pancakes or serve them with mashed potatoes or brown rice. If you choose eggs for breakfast, be sure to have some fresh fruit as well.

Mixed Berry Muesli

You can now use rolled (porridge) oats or rolled barley in muesli, as well as rice flakes.

Ingredients

1 tablespoon raw porridge oats

2 tablespoons of water or fresh fruit juice (apple juice is excellent)

150 g of fresh berries, including raspberries, strawberries, blackberries, black currants, mulberries, etc.

rice milk or oat milk

Method

Place the oats in a bowl and add the water or juice. Pile the berries on top, add rice or oat milk and serve.

Winter Muesli

Ingredients

1 tablespoon raw rolled barley
1 tablespoon oat bran
1/2 apple, chopped

1/2 pear, chopped
1/2 banana, chopped
rice milk or oat milk

Method

Place the barley and bran in a bowl and soften in a small amount of the rice milk. Add the chopped fruit (peel the apple and pear unless they are organically grown) and serve with rice or oat milk.

Scrambled Eggs with Onion and Rice

Ingredients

virgin olive oil
1 onion, finely chopped
2 eggs
fresh chives, chopped

salt and pepper to taste
pre-cooked brown rice, heated in
　　boiling water and then strained

Method

Warm the olive oil, add the onion and cook until soft.
Beat the eggs lightly, add most of the chives, and seasoning.
Add the beaten eggs to the onions and cook until the eggs are firm but still soft.
Serve on the rice, decorate with remaining chives.

Poached Eggs on Mashed Potato

Ingredients

3 small potatoes, diced
virgin olive oil
water or vegetable stock

2 eggs
salt and white pepper to taste
paprika

Method

Cook the diced potato until soft, mash, adding a small amount of olive oil and sufficient water or vegetable stock to achieve the desired consistency. Season to taste.
Poach the eggs in boiling water or in poaching pans over boiling water.
Serve the eggs on a bed of mashed potato, decorated with a fine sprinkle of paprika.

Sautéed Eggs on Hash Browns

This is an American dish and is normally made with a lot of fat, so is not good for the liver. However, if you are conservative with the oil, you can still make a meal that is both delicious and healthy.

Ingredients

2 teaspoons olive oil

2 potatoes, grated

1 red onion, finely chopped

2 eggs

salt and pepper to taste

Method

Warm the olive oil in a heavy-based frying pan. Add the chopped onion and cook until transparent. Add the grated potato and cook over a medium heat, turning frequently. Season to taste and keep hot.

Add just enough olive oil to the pan to prevent sticking, break in the eggs and cook gently until done to the required degree. Do not let the oil smoke or the egg whites become browned.

Serve the eggs either on or beside the hash browns.

Spanish Omelette

Ingredients (serves three)

1 teaspoon virgin olive oil

1 onion, finely chopped

1 green and 1 red pepper, finely chopped

3 cooked potatoes, diced

a few leftover vegetables if available

6 eggs

salt and pepper to taste

Method

Warm the olive oil and sauté the chopped onion and peppers until soft.

Add the diced potatoes and any other cooked vegetables and stir.

Beat the 6 eggs lightly together, season and pour them over the vegetables, stirring so the mixture penetrates them.

When cooked on the base, turn the omelette over, carefully, and cook the other side.

Serve with cooked potatoes or brown rice as these make a good balance to the richness of the eggs.

Kedgeree

Kedgeree is traditionally made from leftover rice and fish with the addition of chopped hard-boiled eggs and mustard to season, so it is ideal for this week. It is also easy and quick to make, provided the ingredients are indeed left over (i.e. already cooked and available).

Ingredients per person

100 g cooked brown rice
50 g cooked fish, flaked
1 hard-boiled egg, shelled and
    chopped
virgin olive oil

English mustard powder to taste
seasoning
sprigs of fresh parsley to
    garnish

Method

Mix dry ingredients together in a bowl (except the parsley and oil).
Warm the olive oil in a skillet.
Add to the skillet and stir-fry until heated through.
Serve garnished with parsley.

Bubble and Squeak

Any leftover vegetables can be reheated in this way and the dish can be served on its own or with eggs. If you have some fish handy this can be added to provide protein.

Ingredients

Leftover or pre-cooked vegetables
    *(Ideally some of them should
    be root vegetables or pumpkin;
    others should be 'wetter'
    vegetables such as cabbage,*

*leeks or tomatoes to provide
    textural variety.)*
virgin olive oil
pre-cooked fish (optional)

Method

Mash or chop the vegetables and mix together.
Warm the oil in a frying pan, add the mixed vegetables and heat through, turning frequently to avoid burning. If you are going to include fish, add it towards the end to avoid breaking it up.

Basic Pancakes

Pancakes can make an excellent substitute for bread.

Ingredients

140 g barley flour   250 ml rice milk
2 eggs, separated   virgin olive oil

Method

Combine 200 ml of the rice milk with the barley flour. Add the beaten yolks to the flour and rice milk and mix well. Beat the whites until stiff and fold into the mixture. Add more rice milk until the desired consistency is obtained.

Lightly oil a hot skillet and pour in sufficient batter to cover the base. Cook until bubbles form and the batter can be lifted from the pan. Turn and cook on the other side. Lift out onto a plate.

Variations

Pancakes can be made with other types of flour, such as oat flour, buckwheat flour, rice flour or a combination. They are generally more fragile and may not roll up as well as when made with barley flour, in which case use them for the small and stiffer pikelets. Adding an extra egg can improve their strength.

Week 5

The pancakes can be made with wheat flour.

Pikelets

Use the Basic Pancake mixture *(see above)*, but make the mixture thicker by decreasing the amount of liquid. Add only one spoonful of batter to the pan such that it spreads out to about 5–7 cm in diameter. Several can be cooked in the pan at one time.

Storing Pancakes

Pancakes and pikelets can be made ahead of time and stored ready for use. Make them in the normal way. Place alternating pancakes and layers of greaseproof paper in a stack, wrap in a tea towel and store in the refrigerator.

Serving Suggestions

- Serve with fresh fruit, including from such recipes as Mixed Berry and Mint Delight, Winter Special or Spicy Fruit Salad.

- Use pancakes as a base for egg dishes, instead of toast.
- Fill them with leftovers from dinner the night before, roll them up, wrap firmly in greaseproof paper and take them to work for lunch.

Vegetable Fritter/Pancakes

Ingredients
Basic Pancake batter   virgin olive oil
leftover vegetables

Method
Add the leftover vegetables to the pancake batter, making sure there is sufficient batter to hold the fritters together.
Cook small amounts in a lightly oiled hot skillet until cooked and browned on both sides.
Can also be used to replace sandwiches, at lunch time.

Week 5

As this is still part of your detox plan, make sure most of your breakfasts are based on fresh fruit or perhaps some vegetables. However the following recipes will provide added variety. They are also appropriate, in combination with fresh fruit, if you are doing heavy physical activity.

Hungry Muesli

In this week's version of muesli there is greater emphasis on different types of grains than before and the inclusion of nuts and seeds. Keep in mind, however, that this should continue to be essentially a fruit dish.

Ingredients
50 g each of rolled oats, rolled   50 g of linseeds
   barley, wheat germ, rice bran   50 g lecithin granules
50 g mixed chopped raw nuts,   fresh fruit
   choose from cashews, almonds,
   brazils, and sunflower seeds

Method
Combine the dry ingredients, mix well and store in an airtight container. Do not be tempted to make larger quantities unless several people will be eating it.

Per serving
Put 1 heaped tablespoon of the dry mixture in a bowl, soften with warm water or fruit juice. Add chopped fresh fruit, approximately the equivalent of 2 large apples. Serve with rice milk, oat milk or fruit juice.

Variation
Omit the nuts and seeds from the dry mixture, instead sprinkle them over the top of each dish as decoration.

Eggs
All the egg dishes from Week 3 can be used and you can serve them with pancakes. Try to have dishes that include vegetables. These could include omelettes and scrambled eggs with a wide variety of vegetables, either hot or cold, and either incorporated into the dish or served beside it. Have some fresh fruit as well, to balance the meal.

Pancakes
Pancakes can now be made with wheat flour if you prefer, but by this stage you may be enjoying the flavours of the different grains

The Future

Now that some dairy products can be included you can serve the muesli dishes with plain yoghurt. You can have wholemeal bread with the eggs and other dishes. It would be better to use olive oil rather than butter as a spread, do not use margarine and avoid the temptation to have sugar-laden jams and marmalades. However you can have some of the sugar-free jams that are available from health food shops, sweetened or made with fruit juice instead of sugar.

If you want a substantial breakfast it would still be wise to include vegetables and fresh fruit. So include such dishes as grilled tomatoes or mushrooms on toast, or Bubble and Squeak with toast.

Original Muesli

Muesli, as originally developed and used in many of the early health clinics in Europe, was essentially a fruit dish. The fruit provides flavour, sweetness, vitamins and a cleansing and alkalising effect; the oats (or other grain) are digested slowly and help to keep your blood sugar level up, as well as providing minerals and vitamins; the yoghurt provides protein (which combines well with the protein in the grains) as well as calcium; and the nuts or seeds provide essentially fatty acids, something firm to chew and flavour. This is an extremely healthy breakfast and can be varied endlessly, so need never be boring.

Ingredients per person

1 tablespoon rolled oats	2–3 tablespoons plain yoghurt
water, fruit juice or milk	1 tablespoon sunflower seeds
1 apple, finely chopped	1 tablespoon lecithin granules
1 pear, finely chopped	

Method

Place the oats in a bowl and moisten with the liquid. Add the lecithin granules, then chopped fresh fruit and the yoghurt, decorate with the sunflower seeds.

Variations

Replace the oats with other grains, or combinations of grains.

Replace the apple and pear with any other combination of fresh fruit you can think of.

Replace the sunflower seeds with chopped raw nuts (not peanuts).

Instead of layering the dish, mix all ingredients in a bowl before serving.

———— Snacks, Nibbles and Starters ————

Week 1

Starters

Many cold, lightly cooked, vegetables make an excellent start to a meal. A mixture of broccoli and cauliflower provides colour variation. You will think of others for yourself. Toss them in an olive oil and lemon dressing and serve on a bed of greens or in a scooped out orange half or prepared sweet pepper. Garnish with fresh herbs.

Artichoke hearts or, in season, lightly cooked fresh asparagus, are delicious. Simply use olive oil instead of butter (until you reach The Future, when conservative use of dairy products is permitted).

Half a grapefruit makes an excellent start to a meal. Pick one of the pink grapefruit and you won't need sugar. Eat as much of the pith as you can, for the beneficial bioflavonoids that benefit the liver.

Any of the salads can be used as starters – simply reduce the quantities and serve elegantly on a bed of leaves. Alternatively you can simply arrange a few vegetable pieces on a plate, such as alternating slices of cucumber and radish, or sticks of celery and carrot with a light dressing from the selection for Week 1.

Crudités

Ingredients

salad dressing of your choice
(see p.104)

raw vegetables such as carrots,
    cucumber, courgette, celery,
    broccoli, cauliflower

alfalfa sprouts

Method

Place the salad dressing in a small bowl and put the bowl in the centre
of a large plate.

Slice the vegetables or cut into bite-sized pieces and arrange around the
bowl of salad dressing. Surround with alfalfa sprouts. Dip the vegetables into the dressing and enjoy.

Artichokes, Plain

You may think of artichoke as a luxury food, but remember the benefits
it can confer on your liver and eat it often.

Ingredients

1 artichoke per person   virgin olive oil

Method

Rinse the artichokes thoroughly, in salty water. Open the leaves slightly
so anything that is trapped there can be flushed away. Place in water
and boil for about 30 minutes or until an outer leaf comes away readily
when pulled, and the thick base of the leaf is tender. Drain and cool.

To eat, pull off each leaf and use your teeth to pull the fleshy base away
from the fibrous leaf. When all the leaves have been dealt with in this way
remove the 'choke', the fibrous clump on top of the heart, and eat the latter.

Variations

Dip each leaf into a drop of virgin olive oil.

Artichoke with Herb Dressing

Ingredients

artichokes, prepared as above
1 small clove garlic, crushed
    (optional)
1 teaspoon finely chopped fresh
    herbs (oregano, marjoram, basil,
    chervil, parsley, tarragon, etc.)

1 teaspoon chopped fresh chives
salt and freshly ground black-
    pepper
3 tablespoons virgin olive oil
1 tablespoon fresh lemon juice
    (to taste)

Method
Combine the garlic, herbs and seasoning and blend into a smooth paste.
Add the lemon juice and work it in, then do the same with the oil.

Variations
In The Future: Use a 50:50 mixture of butter (melted) and olive oil. Use
wine vinegar in place of some of the lemon juice. Add 1 teaspoon capers,
chopped.

Artichoke Hearts

Because artichokes are so good for your liver, using tinned artichoke
hearts, as a convenience and when you are short of time, could be an
acceptable 'cheat'.
    Arrange them on a bed of lettuce leaves and serve with a dressing of
your choice (see p.104).

Beetroot with Chives

Ingredients
1 teaspoon virgin olive oil
1/2 teaspoon fresh lemon juice
4 beetroot, cooked, peeled and
    sliced (very good for your liver)

a generous bunch of chives,
    chopped

Method
Combine the oil and lemon juice, pour over the beetroot, add the chives
and toss. Serve on a bed of lettuce leaves.

Prawn Cocktail

This is a perennial favourite and can easily be incorporated into your
diet even at this early stage.

Ingredients
prawns, either fresh or frozen
your choice of vegetable for
    display purposes
*(You might, for instance, choose
simply to arrange the prawns on a
bed of lettuce; alternatively, scoop
out a cucumber and pile the
prawns into the centre; or lightly*

*steam an onion cut in half cross-
ways, scoop out the centre and fill;
or cut lengths of leeks about 10 cm
long and carefully peel out the
centre and arrange the prawns
inside.)*
dressing of your choice (see p.104)
lemon wedges

Method

Mix the prawns with your chosen dressing. Arrange the vegetable on small plate, pile in the prawns and serve decorated with wedges of lemon.

Variation

A flaked fish cocktail can be made in the same way as a prawn cocktail but using cooked fish instead of the prawns. Flake the fish, toss in the dressing and arrange on or in a bed of vegetables.

Week 3

Continue to select starters from the recipes above but you can now also choose from the following recipes.

Now that you can eat eggs and make mayonnaise you can include starters such as egg mayonnaise and the ubiquitous prawn cocktail with real mayonnaise (instead of having to choose an egg-free dressing), or prawns in an avocado shell. Salads continue to make an excellent start to a meal and you can be a bit more adventurous with them now too, including tomatoes and peppers, for instance.

Crudités with Avocado Dip

Ingredients

1 large ripe avocado, mashed
1 lemon, juiced

cayenne pepper and salt to taste
vegetable pieces (as crudités p.93)

Method

Combine the avocado, lemon juice and seasoning, mix thoroughly and pile into a bowl. Place on a platter, surrounded by the vegetable pieces.

Eggs with Caviar

This is a treat, use it when entertaining.

Ingredients

4 eggs, hard boiled
50 g caviar
$1/4$ lemon
1 tablespoon basic mayonnaise

salt and pepper
lettuce leaves and cucumber slices
    to decorate

Method

Cut the eggs in half length-ways and scoop out the yolks. Fill the egg whites with caviar and squeeze a few drops of lemon juice over it. Mash the egg yolks with the mayonnaise, season, and spread over the whites arranged on a bed of lettuce leaves and surrounded by cucumber slices.

Grilled Asparagus

You can, of course, simply steam the asparagus and serve it with virgin olive oil, instead of butter as you did in Week 1. However this is an interesting variation.

Ingredients

1 bunch asparagus trimmed
2 tablespoons virgin olive oil
1 egg, hard boiled
1 tablespoon freshly squeezed
   lemon juice

1 teaspoon chervil or dill, finely
   chopped
2 spring onions, finely chopped

Method

Lay the asparagus on a plate, brush with a little of the olive oil and grill slowly until tender.

Meanwhile, mash the egg, add olive oil and mix to a smooth paste, add the lemon juice, herbs and spring onions and mix thoroughly.

Season to taste.

Pour the sauce over the cooked asparagus and serve.

Week 5

Crudités should still be a frequent choice when you want a snack or something to nibble on before a meal. You can now include a dish of raw nuts or sunflower seeds. Toasted Sunflower Seeds *(see below)* can add variety.

Toasted Sunflower Seeds

Ingredients

1 teaspoon olive oil
1 teaspoon of mixed spices of your
   choice (choose from cumin,

coriander, cardamom, cayenne
   pepper, etc.)
150 g sunflower seeds

Method

Warm the oil in a skillet, add the spices and stir until smooth. Add the sunflower seeds and stir until well coated. Continue to cook, stirring occasionally, until the seeds have browned.

Variation

Follow the same recipe using raw nuts instead. Almonds are particularly good.

In The Future

Add a tablespoon of soy sauce towards the end of cooking.

Spiced Seeds and Nuts

Ingredients

100 g each of almonds, brazil nuts, cashews, hazelnuts, pine kernels and sunflower seeds
If you have strong preferences use greater amounts of the nuts of your choice. You can use walnuts, but be warned, you may get unexpected 'pockets' of spices caught in the crevices that can be somewhat overwhelming! Do not use peanuts. All the nuts must be raw and should not have been chopped or broken.

5 tablespoons virgin olive oil
1 teaspoon mild chilli powder (to taste)
1 teaspoon paprika
1 teaspoon ground coriander
1 teaspoon ground cumin
$1/2$ teaspoon ground cardamom
$1/4$ teaspoon ground fenugreek
$1/4$ teaspoon ground allspice
$1/4$ teaspoon ground ginger
$1/2$ teaspoon grated nutmeg

Method

Spread the nuts and seeds on a tray and bake in the oven at 200°C for about five minutes, stirring frequently, until they are lightly browned but not burnt. Heat the olive oil in a heavy skillet, add the spices and cook for a few minutes, then add the nuts and mix thoroughly.

You can add salt if you must, but the mixture is tasty as it is. As you experiment you can vary both the nuts and the spices to suit your taste. Store in an airtight container and have some with you at times when you might want a snack.

Chick Peas

Chick peas, also known as garbonzo beans, are an excellent source of protein with a delicate flavour of peas, rather than beans.

Nahit

Ingredients

300 g chick peas
freshly ground black pepper

salt and pepper

Method

Soak the chick peas in warm water overnight. Drain, cover with more water and soak for another 24 hours. By this time tiny shoots should be showing at the 'tip' of the seeds and they should be soft enough to eat raw. Drain the peas and roll in the salt and pepper while still wet. Serve as a snack in place of peanuts or crisps.

Variation
Add cayenne pepper and other spices, such as cumin and coriander to the salt and pepper. Be careful if you use paprika or turmeric, as the colour may spoil your clothes.
Use the prepared chick peas instead of nuts in the previous recipe.

Chick Pea Savouries

Ingredients
250 g chick pea flour
1 teaspoon turmeric (very good for your liver)
1/2 teaspoon ground cumin
1/2 teaspoon ground cardamom
1/2 teaspoon allspice

1/4 teaspoon chilli powder (to taste)
3 eggs, separated
2–3 large cloves garlic, crushed
water or vegetable stock
virgin olive oil for frying

Method
Combine the dry ingredients. Add the egg yolks and garlic and just sufficient liquid to make a smooth paste. Whip the whites until stiff and fold into the mixture. Drop spoonfuls onto a lightly oiled heavy-based skillet and heat until the base is cooked. Turn and cook the other side. Put on kitchen paper to remove excess fat, allow to cool and serve. These also make a convenient snack to take with you when 'on the move'.

The Future

Crudités
There will be many times when you are looking for something to nibble before a meal. Avoid temptation by not purchasing such fat-laden foods as crisps or roast nuts. Instead, prepare some of the nibbles suggested here and have them ready for when they are wanted. Get into the habit of relying on pieces of vegetable rather than high-fat foods.

You can now use yoghurt, crème fraîche or ricotta cheese, in combination with salad dressing, to make dips to serve with crudités. The following are some examples:

- Add a bunch of chives, chopped, and a teaspoon of paprika to a carton of plain yoghurt and stir.
- Combine ricotta cheese with mashed avocado and lemon juice, to taste.
- Mix an equal amount of French dressing or mayonnaise with plain yoghurt.

Soups

When making the stocks described below the aim is to extract all the flavours and minerals you can from the solid ingredients, which you will then, generally, be discarding.

Once you have added the fresh ingredients to the pot they should be cooked briefly, just long enough to make them tender. One of the biggest mistakes that is generally made in regard to soups is overcooking.

Week 1

Basic Stock

This is a basic vegetable stock that you can use as the liquid in any of the recipes below or that you can use in your own recipes. It helps to add the flavours you might in the past have got from stock cubes; these you now have to avoid, as they will probably contain yeast and other ingredients you should not have, at least for the moment. It is also economical as you can use the parts of vegetables that you might otherwise throw away.

If you feel that making this is too much trouble, you can simply use water in recipes that call for stock, but you might then want to add additional fresh herbs.

Ingredients
fish bones (if available) (optional)
fresh lemon juice
any vegetable trimmings
(These can be any trimmings that you might otherwise throw away, such as celery tops, the outer stalks from a bunch of celery, the leaves from cauliflower and broccoli, the outer leaves of cabbage or lettuce, beetroot greens and so forth. You can also use 'old' vegetables that are tired and no longer appealing to serve as fresh vegetables.)

Method
Place the bones in sufficient water to cover them, add the lemon juice, bring to the boil and simmer for one to two hours. By adding the lemon juice you increase the chance of leaching some of the minerals, such as calcium and magnesium, out of the bones.

Chop the vegetables, add and simmer for another 30 minutes.

Allow to stand for two hours, strain, discard the solids and store the liquid in the refrigerator.

Use within a day or two, alternatively freeze the liquid until needed.

If you wish to have a thick soup, use rice flour for thickening.

Sweet Onion Soup

Ingredients
virgin olive oil
3 large onions, peeled and diced
1 clove garlic, finely chopped
1 small apple, grated
Basic Stock or water

fresh herb leaves as available
(oregano or marjoram are
excellent)
salt and freshly ground black-
pepper to taste

Method
Sauté the onions and garlic in sufficient oil to prevent sticking, until soft and golden. Add the grated apple, stir and cook for two minutes.
Add the herbs and then the stock or water, bring to the boil and simmer for 10 minutes.
Season and serve, decorated with some of the fresh herb leaves.

Mediterranean Fish Soup

Strictly speaking this recipe should include white wine, but since you cannot have that yet I have substituted the lemon juice (for the tang) and the coriander (for flavour).

Ingredients
500 g mixed fish and shellfish
1 litre water or vegetable stock
juice of 1 lemon
2 bay leaves
1 tablespoon olive oil

1 large onion, diced
2 small cloves garlic, chopped
2 sticks celery, chopped
1 tablespoon chopped parsley
1/2 tablespoon chopped coriander

Method
Prepare the fish and shellfish. Put the bones, shells and skins in the water, with the lemon juice and bay leaves, simmer for 30 minutes, strain and discard the solids. Heat the olive oil in a heavy-based skillet and sauté the onion and garlic until soft and golden. Add the chopped celery and herbs, then the fish and shellfish, stir for a few minutes, add the stock, stir, simmer for 30 minutes, season before serving.

Bouillabaisse

After cooking this dish you'll know that a cleansing diet need not be time-consuming to prepare or dull to the taste buds. Reduce the quantities if appropriate.

Ingredients

6 cloves of garlic, crushed
2 large onions, chopped
2 sticks celery, finely chopped
5 tablespoons olive oil
1 tablespoon parsley, chopped
1 bay leaf
1 tablespoon chopped fresh dill
    or 1 teaspoon chopped fresh
    fennel leaves

100 g each of cod, halibut, bream,
    monk fish, turbot, whiting (or
    600 g of mixed fish), cut into
    bite-sized pieces
the meat of one small lobster
100 g crab meat
100 g prawns, shelled
water or stock

Method

Place all the ingredients in a saucepan, warm gently. Cover with boiling water or stock and simmer for 15 minutes. The amount of water you add will depend on whether you want to serve this as a soup or a main dish.

Variation

Week 3: Include 3 or 4 chopped tomatoes and one sliced green pepper.

Week 3

Basic Stock

Follow the recipe for Basic Stock in Week 1, but you can now use the bones of chicken and other poultry as well as or instead of fish.
You can now use barley flour to thicken a soup, if desired.

Bouillabaisse

See variation to the Bouillabaisse recipe above.

Fish Soup with Paprika

Ingredients

500 g fish
2 teaspoons sweet paprika
1/2 teaspoon salt

2 onions, chopped
1 red and 1 green pepper, chopped

Method

Cut the flesh of the fish off the bone and separate it from the skin. Make a stock by simmering the bones plus the paprika and salt in 1 litre of water for 30 minutes, strain.

Meanwhile cut the fish into small pieces, combine with the chopped onions and pepper, add to the stock and simmer until fish and vegetables are cooked.

Sweet Pepper Soup

Ingredients

1 red pepper, 1 green pepper, 1 yellow pepper and 1 orange pepper

5 ml virgin olive oil

1 Spanish onion, diced

2 cloves garlic, chopped

500 ml vegetable stock

sprig fresh marjoram and oregano

Method

Roast the peppers in a hot oven (220°C) for half an hour. Allow to cool slightly, peel and chop finely.

Warm the olive oil in a heavy-based saucepan and sauté the onion and garlic, slowly, over a medium heat until transparent. Add the chopped peppers and toss. Add the marjoram and stock and simmer for 10 minutes or until the peppers are very soft.

Serve decorated with fresh sprigs of oregano.

Chicken Soup

Ingredients

1 chicken carcass

vegetables as available, e.g.
  1 carrot, grated; 1 parsnip, grated; 1 onion, finely chopped;

celery leaves, chopped;

1 pepper, finely chopped;

1 small leek, finely chopped.

Salt and pepper

Method

Simmer the chicken carcass for one hour in sufficient water to cover it. Strain, add the vegetables to the stock and simmer for about 10 minutes. Season, serve as it is, or homogenise the soup in a blender, reheat and serve.

Variations

If you have time, allow the chicken stock to cool and remove the fat that solidifies on the surface. Reheat and continue.

For a more satisfying soup add a handful of barley to the strained stock, simmer until cooked, then add the vegetables and continue.

Egg Soup

Ingredients

3 egg yolks (*no* whites)
1 litre Basic Stock *(p.101)*

2–4 tablespoons pre-cooked (or leftover) vegetables, fish or chicken, chopped

Method

Beat the egg yolks and add a small amount of the stock. Continue to beat and gradually add the rest of the stock.

Heat in a double boiler, stirring constantly. It will gradually start to thicken. When it has, add the vegetables, fish or chicken, heat through, season to taste and serve.

Week 5

You will now be able to use many soups in your recipe books. Simply use oat or rice milk instead of cow's milk. For a creamier texture use olive oil instead of cream (if you haven't already tried this you may be in for a pleasant surprise). If your own recipes contain ingredients you cannot yet eat, find substitutes. Be patient, The Future is not far away.

Basic Stock

Now that red meat is included in your diet you can use a variety of meat bones as well as poultry and fish, to make a soup stock. If you still feel that making this is too much trouble then you can simply use water, but remember to add additional fresh herbs if you want an interesting flavour.

Ingredients

meat, chicken, fish or other bones as available
fresh lemon juice
any vegetable trimmings *(such as the outer stalks or tops from a bunch of celery, the leaves from cauliflower and broccoli, the outer leaves of cabbage or lettuce, beetroot greens and so forth. You can also use 'old' vegetables that are no longer appealing to serve as fresh vegetables.)*

Method

Place the bones in sufficient water to cover them, add the lemon juice, bring to the boil and simmer for one to two hours. By adding the lemon juice you increase the chance of leaching some of the minerals, such as calcium and magnesium, out of the bones.

Chop the vegetables, add and simmer for another 30 minutes.
Allow to stand for two hours, strain, discard the solids and store the liquid in the refrigerator.
Use within a day or two or freeze once cooled.

The Future

Soups will continue to have a place in your diet and the ones you make at home will be much better than those you buy in tins or cartons. Base them on stock you have made yourself, meat, fish and fresh vegetables with herbs and spices for seasoning. With a little ingenuity you will be able to use or adapt (and make more nutritious) many of the recipes you already have. Use wholemeal flour instead of white flour or corn flour, for thickening, for instance, and replace cream or sour cream with plain yoghurt.

Salad Dressings

Fresh vegetables should be a major component of your diet and a large proportion of them should be eaten raw, as salads. Ideally, you should have a salad for lunch each day and a side salad for dinner. To add interest you may want to experiment with a number of different salad dressings. Use them in moderation, however, not to swamp the dish. I recall in one American restaurant being given what looked like a bowl of mayonnaise with a few lettuce leaves floating in it – not good!

Week 1

Lemon Juice or Vinegar
At the start of the Liver Detox Plan you cannot have vinegar, nor can you have it until such time as you are sure that you do not have a problem with candida. For this reason the juice of lemon, lime or other fruit is used with oil to make the salad dressings, at least until The Future. All the dressings should be stored in the refrigerator. Not only does this keep the oil fresh, but it is necessary as they are made with fruit juices, fresh herbs or vegetables.

The Oil
You will generally use virgin olive oil but for variety and by Week 5 this can be replace by others, such as walnut oil, almond oil or apricot kernel oil. Buy these oils in small bottles and use quickly once opened to avoid the dangers of rancidity. Avoid the commercial cooking or salad oils such as peanut oil, corn oil, soy oil, etc., as the processing leads to an oil with undesirable characteristics.

Lecithin
Adding lecithin granules to the dressing will benefit your liver and will also add an interesting variation to the texture as the liquid (lemon juice now, vinegar later) and oil will remain mixed instead of separating on standing. If you use lecithin it is best to make only as much as you plan to use. Remember, your aim is to have a total of 1 tablespoon of lecithin granules a day.

Lemon French Dressing

Ingredients

1 tablespoon fresh lemon juice

3 tablespoons virgin olive oil

1 teaspoon lecithin granules (optional)

small clove of garlic, crushed

Method
Combine all ingredients in a jar, shake well and store in the refrigerator.

Variation
Replace the lemon juice with lime or grapefruit juice.

English–French Dressing

Ingredients

1 tablespoons fresh lemon juice

3 tablespoons virgin olive oil

1/4 teaspoon English mustard powder

salt and freshly ground black-pepper to taste

Method
Combine all ingredients in a jar, shake well and store in the refrigerator.

Herb Dressing

Ingredients

1 tablespoon fresh lemon juice

3 tablespoons virgin olive oil

1 teaspoon lecithin granules (optional)

1 tablespoon chopped fresh herbs; choose from basil, dill, oregano, parsley, chervil and coriander

salt and freshly ground black-pepper

Method
Combine all ingredients, mix well and stored in an airtight container in the refrigerator.

This is a large quantity of herbs, but you will not be having many of the flavourings you are used to and the herbs are an excellent substitute. Use less if you prefer.

Lime and Pepper Dressing

Ingredients

3 tablespoons virgin olive oil
1 tablespoon fresh lime juice
1 teaspoon lecithin granules
  (optional)

2 cloves garlic, crushed
freshly ground black pepper
1 pinch sea salt

Method

Combine all ingredients and store in the refrigerator.

Oil-Free Dressing

Ingredients

1 tablespoon fresh lemon
  juice
4 tablespoons fresh apple
  juice
1/4 cucumber, peeled (even if it is
  organically grown)

1/2 tablespoon chopped fresh dill
  or 1 teaspoonful chopped fresh
  fennel weed
1 clove garlic, crushed
salt and freshly ground black
  pepper

Method

Place all ingredients in a blender and blend until smooth. Keep refrigerated.

Banana Mayonnaise

You cannot, at this time, use eggs and make true mayonnaise, but this is a possible alternative.

Ingredients

French dressing   ripe banana(s)

Method

Place the ingredients in a blender and blend until smooth. If you do not have a blender, mash the banana thoroughly and mix well.
Adjust the proportions to suit your taste.

Week 3

Continue to choose dressings from the above recipes, but now that eggs are included you can make mayonnaise as well – and you probably *will* have to make it yourself as commercial ones generally contain vinegar.

Basic Mayonnaise

Make this in a blender if you have one. If not, use an egg whisk, but this is hard work.

Ingredients
2 egg yolks
1/2 teaspoon English mustard
   powder
1/4 teaspoon salt

2 tablespoons freshly squeezed
   lemon juice
200 ml virgin olive oil

Method
Blend the egg yolks, mustard, salt and lemon juice.
Keep the blender running and add the oil very gradually, drop by drop initially and then in a slightly faster, intermittent drizzle. The aim is to make sure that each addition of oil has combined with the mixture before adding more. If you get impatient and fail to do this your mayonnaise may separate and you will have to start over again.

Variations
Use lime or grapefruit juice instead of lemon juice. Add herbs or chopped chives. Add paprika to taste.

In The Future
You can replace the lemon juice with vinegar and add a tiny amount of honey.

Pineapple Mayonnaise

This is another blender mayonnaise.

Ingredients
2 egg yolks
2 tablespoons fresh lemon
   juice
1/4 teaspoon salt

2 slices of fresh pineapple, or
   tinned but unsweetened
   pineapple
approximately 200 ml virgin olive
   oil

Method
Blend the eggs, lemon juice, salt and pineapple. Keep the blender running and add the oil drop by drop, then in a slow drizzle as before. Add less or more oil to obtain your favoured consistency.

Variation
Replace the pineapple with any other fruit.

Week 5

You can add variety to dressings by using some of the delicious nut and seed oils that are available. They include almond oil, walnut oil and apricot kernel oil. They are generally more expensive than olive oil, but keep in mind that you are using them for their flavour as well as for their fat content. While you might think you can now use soy, corn or sunflower oil, it is better that you don't. They are much more processed than olive oil and present a greater challenge to your liver, so plan to continue using olive oil as your main oil long term.

The Future

You can now use vinegar in salad dressings instead of lemon juice, if desired. Make sure the vinegar is of good quality and choose from apple cider vinegar, wine vinegar (with or without herbs) or balsamic vinegar. Some types of vinegar, especially the cheap ones, are nothing more than acetic acid and should be avoided.

Mayonnaise

Make this in a blender if you have one. If not, use an egg whisk, but this is hard work.

Ingredients

2 egg yolks
$1/2$ teaspoon English mustard
  powder
$1/4$ teaspoon salt

1 teaspoon liquid honey
2 tablespoons wine vinegar
200 ml virgin olive oil

Method
Blend the egg yolks, mustard, salt, honey and vinegar. Keep the blender running and add the oil very gradually, drop by drop initially and then in a slightly faster, intermittent drizzle. The aim is to make sure that each addition of oil has combined with the mixture before adding more. If you get impatient and fail to do this, your mayonnaise may separate.

Salads

To encourage yourself to increase the amount of vegetables in your diet, refer back to p.25 and reread the benefits specific vegetables offer both to your liver and as part of the Liver Detox Plan. Promise yourself you will include as many as possible in your diet – and certainly a lot more than you have in the past.

Week 1

You will doubtless have your own salad preferences, so use them, provided they consist of fresh fruit and vegetables and don't include potatoes, tomatoes, peppers, aubergine, avocado, mushrooms or pickled vegetables. The ingredients can be combined in an infinite number of ways.

If, in the past, a salad has meant to you a plate containing lettuce, cucumber and tomato with maybe a slice or two of tinned beetroot and a spring onion, this really is the time to expand your thinking. You can eat almost any vegetable raw, especially if you grate or chop it small enough. You can also combine fruit with the vegetables to provide greater interest and variety. A banana, for instance, chopped through a salad, can compensate for not being able to use mayonnaise. Become adventuresome and use vegetables that you may not have thought of in the past. Some ideas are given below.

These recipes are not, of course, intended to be an exhaustive list, nor are they the only ones you can eat. They are given simply to stimulate your imagination.

Just as it was important that you presented your fruit breakfasts with elegance and style, the way you present a salad is important to your soul and your moods as well as to your digestion. There are so many different colours and textures to choose from that you should have no trouble creating meals that look interesting and help your liver as an important part of the Liver Detox Plan.

Side Salads
Whenever possible your lunch and dinner should either consist of or be accompanied by a side salad. If this is not possible then eat a piece of fruit or some vegetable crudités. Any of the salads given below, or any of the ones you can dream up using the ingredients permitted for this week, can be used as a side salad. The choice is yours. Adjust the quantities as appropriate.

Beetroot
Beetroot is particularly good for your liver and should be included in or served with salads whenever possible. Use fresh beetroot, not the tinned variety, as that commonly contains vinegar and sugar as well as possible other additives.

Beetroot can be eaten raw, in which case it should be cleaned, peeled and grated, but you may also want to cook it. To prepare it, clean the beetroot, cut off the leaves (wash and keep them, they make excellent salad leaves), put the whole beetroot in boiling water and cook until tender. Allow to cool and then peel. Slice and serve will other salad vegetables.

Beetroot Salad

Ingredients

3 raw beetroot, grated
fresh lemon or apple juice

lettuce leaves
a few sprigs of parsley

Method
Combine the grated beetroot and lemon juice. Serve on a bed of lettuce leaves for an interesting colour contrast and decorate with fresh parsley.

Wimbledon Salad

Ingredients

4 large beetroot, cooked, peeled
  and diced
150 g peas, lightly cooked
85 g brown rice, cooked

salad dressing of your choice
  (optional)
watercress for decorating

Method
Combine all ingredients except the parsley, toss well together, pile into a bowl and decorate with the watercress.

Radish Salad

Ingredients

red radishes, grated
Lemon French dressing

lettuce

Method
Toss the radishes in the dressing and arrange on lettuce leaves.

Parsnip Salad

Ingredients

fresh parsnips, peeled and grated
freshly squeezed lemon juice

watercress

Method
Combine the grated parsnip and lemon juice, adjusting the proportions to suit your taste. Decorate with watercress.
This is a surprisingly delicious salad.

Beetroot, Carrot and Parsnip Salad

The interest of this dish lies in the combination of colours. If you have a coarse grater or shredder, use that and the final dish will show the distinctly different colours of the ingredients.

Ingredients
1 raw beetroot, grated
1 carrot, grated
1 parsnip, grated
oil and lemon juice dressing

one or two radishes, finely
 chopped
1 small bunch chives, chopped

Method
Combine the grated vegetables and dressing. Mix lightly (keeping the colours somewhat separate) and place in a salad bowl. Decorate with the chopped radishes and chives.

Mock Coleslaw

Ingredients
1 small sweet white cabbage
1 carrot, grated
2 red-skinned apples (organically
 grown if you are to use the
 skins), grated

1 bunch of fresh chives, chopped,
 keep some for decoration
Banana Mayonnaise
alfalfa sprouts to decorate

Method
Remove the large outer cabbage leaves, clean and set aside, finely chop the rest of the cabbage.
Combine with the rest of the ingredients and serve in a deep bowl, lined with a 'nest' of the outer cabbage leaves. Decorate with a generous quantity of alfalfa sprouts.

Sweet Onion Salad

Unless you like the full flavour of raw onions, choose red onions for this dish, or ones you know to have a mild flavour. If possible, prepare the dish an hour ahead of the meal.

Ingredients
onions
oranges

watercress to decorate

Method
Slice the onions very thinly and lay them in a shallow dish. Juice the oranges and pour the juice over the onions, leaving them to soak for an hour or even more. Decorate with watercress leaves.

Carrot, Cauliflower, Peas and Beans Salad

Ingredients
1 carrot, grated
1/4 head of small cauliflower, chopped finely
50 g peas, lightly cooked but still firm
50 g green beans, lightly cooked but still firm
dressing of your choice

Method
Combine all ingredients and serve on a bed of leaves.

Broccoli and Cauliflower Salad

Ingredients
cauliflower
broccoli
oil and lemon juice dressing
fresh dill weed

Method
Steam the cauliflower and broccoli until half cooked. Allow to cool. Cut into bite-sized pieces, toss in the dressing and serve, decorated with the dill weed.

Comprehensive Salad

This is as much a demonstration that you can eat almost any vegetable raw as a specific recipe. Simply use whichever of the following ingredients you have in the house and think you would enjoy.

Ingredients
small quantities of the following:
   raw grated carrot, beetroot, parsley or pumpkin; chopped broccoli and cauliflower florets (raw or lightly cooked); slices of leek, celery, courgette, cucumber; shredded cabbage (red and green); grated or
chopped apples, chopped pear, banana or other fruit of your choice; chopped chives, parsley, basil, dill, coriander, mint or other herbs of your choice
dressing of your choice
lettuce leaves and watercress for serving

Method

Combine all ingredients except the lettuce leaves and watercress in a large bowl. Arrange the leaves in or on a serving dish or bowl and pile the Comprehensive Salad on top. Decorate with a few pieces of fresh vegetables or herbs.

Bitter Leaves

No selection of salads would be complete without a salad of bitter leaves. This has the added advantage of being convenient since you can buy bags of prepared leaves in many supermarkets. Simply add your choice of dressings from the above recipes and you have an excellent side salad. Add alfalfa sprouts, sliced cucumber or chopped celery if you wish to make it more elaborate. For the sake of your liver, add watercress, some dandelion leaves if they are available and beetroot leaves you may have set aside.

Week 3

Choose from the salad recipes above but you can now add potato, peppers, tomato and aubergine as well as small amounts of avocado (which is high in fat). The following recipes are included for variety rather than for any specific benefit to your liver.

Tomato and Basil Salad

Ingredients

4 large fresh tomatoes, sliced
1 sweet onion, finely chopped
large bunch basil leaves,
    torn

an oil and lemon juice dressing of
    your choice
salt and freshly ground black
    pepper

Method

Combine all the ingredients. Serve on a flat plate so the tomato slices remain intact.

New Potato Salad

Ingredients

small new potatoes, the smallest
    you can find

fresh mint leaves
Basic Mayonnaise (see p.108)

Method
Boil the potatoes, whole, with fresh mint leaves. Be careful not to over-cook the potatoes, allow to cool and add sufficient mayonnaise to coat each potato lightly.

Week 5

Make sure salads continue to be a major component of your meals. Many suggestions have already been given and you will find recipe books with hundreds of other suggestions. The following salad is added for its benefit to your liver.

Tabbouleh

Many people think of this as being dominantly a wheat dish with some parsley. It is not. It is dominantly parsley salad with some wheat. If you keep this in mind while you are preparing it you are more likely to get the proportions right.

Ingredients

2–3 very large bunches of flat-leaf parsley *(this is the main ingredient of this dish, and is why it is so beneficial at this stage)*

200 g burghul (a type of cracked wheat) or buckwheat

juice of 2 lemons

4 large tomatoes, chopped finely

small bunch of spring onions, finely chopped (optional)

salt and freshly ground black pepper

Cos lettuce leaves, to serve

Method
Wash the parsley thoroughly, remove all stalks and chop finely.
Soak the burghul in the lemon juice for two hours (it should become sufficiently soft that it is not a danger to your teeth).
Combine all ingredients just before serving.
Serve on a bed of lettuce leaves.

The Future

Make sure that you continue to have a salad each day, either for lunch or as a side salad with dinner. You can now use dressings made with vinegar and so can choose from many of the ones that are available commercially. You may even choose to make a salad your main dish for dinner. Do this by increasing the quantities or by having several different salads and combining them with a cold protein dish.

Vegetables

Week 1

Because you may, in the past, have considered vegetables to play only a supporting role in a meal and because they should play a lead role in your Liver Detox Plan, remind yourself, if you need to, of their benefits, be going back to p.25 and rereading it.

The best way to eat vegetables during the initial weeks of the Liver Detox Plan is lightly steamed. All vegetables can be cooked this way. If you have a steamer, place prepared vegetables in the top and boiling water in the bottom so that the vegetables cook in the steam. If you do not have a steamer, but do have a saucepan with a well-fitting lid, put 2–3 cm of water in the saucepan, bring it to the boil, add the vegetables, put the lid on, and allow them to cook in the steam.

Provided you are not using aluminium saucepans (aluminium is a toxic metal and some enters the cooking water, so it should be discarded), you can use the water again. Keep it in the refrigerator and use it next time you steam vegetables, boil rice or make a soup.

The vegetables can then be served either plain or tossed with chopped fresh herbs. Alternatively, add a touch of virgin olive oil; this is an advantage if you want the herbs to stick to the vegetables, but should be omitted if you want to lose weight.

Braised Artichokes

Remember that artichokes are particularly good for your liver, so indulge frequently in this delicious vegetable.

Ingredients
1 large onion, diced

3 cloves garlic, chopped

2 bay leaves

3 tablespoons virgin olive oil

4 large artichokes (cut off stems)

1 tablespoon chopped fresh herbs

1 tablespoon lime juice

200 ml stock

Method
Put the oil, onion, garlic and bay leaves in the base of a casserole dish just large enough to hold the artichokes and place in a preheated oven at 180°C for 10 minutes.

Then place the artichokes in the dish, upright, baste with the olive oil and return to the oven for 10 minutes, after which time add the fresh herbs, lemon juice and stock and cover with the lid.

Return to the oven and allow to simmer for about an hour or until the artichokes are cooked and the liquid almost totally reduced.

Variations

If using dried herbs, add them with the bay leaves.

Add a variety of other vegetables, wedged around the artichokes, to make a more satisfying dish.

Carrots with Parsnips

Ingredients

equal amounts of carrots and
  parsnips
vegetable stock

virgin olive oil
salt and a generous amount of
  white pepper

Method

Cook the carrots and parsnips in boiling water. Strain.

Mash the vegetables and add just sufficient vegetable stock to moisten and sufficient oil to make very slightly creamy.

Season with salt and white pepper.

Winter Vegetables in the Oven

Ingredients

1 red onion, sliced
1 red sweet potato, cut into
  chunks
1/4 small celeriac, peeled and cut
  into chunks the same size as
  the sweet potato chunks
1 parsnip, cut into same sized
  chunks

1 carrot, cut into same sized
  chunks
5 ml freshly squeezed lemon or
  lime juice
5 ml virgin olive oil
salt and freshly ground black
  pepper to taste

Method

Lay the onion slices over the base of a casserole dish, there is no need to oil it.

Arrange the vegetable chunks on top of the onion slices.

Combine the lemon juice, oil and seasoning and pour over the vegetables.

Put the lid on the casserole dish and bake the vegetables at 180° until tender.

The length of time will depend on the sizes of the chunks but should be around 45 minutes.

Remove the lid for the last 10 minutes, basting the vegetables with the liquid in the dish.

Layered Vegetables

This is a simpler dish than the Winter Vegetables above and preserves all the flavours of the vegetables much better than steaming.

Ingredients

onions and/or leeks plus whatever vegetables you have available

fresh herbs in sprigs

Method

Slice the onions and/or leeks and cover the base of a casserole dish. These vegetables will 'sweat' sufficiently to prevent sticking. Cut the other vegetables into sizes such that they will all cook in the same length of time. This means thin slices of root vegetables and large wedges of cauliflower for instance. Layer these vegetables on the onions and lay sprigs of fresh herbs on top. Put the lid on and bake at 150°C for about 45 minutes or until cooked.

Sweet Potatoes with Mint and Chives

You will not be eating potatoes just yet, but these provide an interesting and satisfying alternative.

Ingredients

500 g white sweet potatoes
2 ml virgin olive oil

generous sprigs of mint, leaves chopped
bunch of chives, chopped

Method

Peel and boil the sweet potatoes until tender. Drain, chop, add the olive oil and toss until the sweet potatoes are coated. Add the chopped mint and chives and toss until well mixed. Serve hot or cold. Cold the potatoes can be made into a delicate sweet potato salad by adding a small amount of mayonnaise.

Stuffed Vegetables

You can stuff a variety of vegetables, so the following 'recipe' is more a series of suggestions than specific instructions.

Ingredients for the stuffing

(quantities will depend on what you are stuffing, your own taste and pre-ferences, so the following is a guide)
fresh garlic, onions and a combination of other vegetables *(keep the stuffing*

relatively firm and dry by using a high proportion of root or starchy vegetables)
fresh herbs for flavour
fish (optional)
olive oil

Method
Chop then sauté the onions and garlic in olive oil.
Chop the other vegetables (including the edible parts scooped out of the container vegetable(s) (below) and set aside) and steam until tender.
Cook the fish (if using it).
Chop the herbs.
Combine all these ingredients and use as stuffing for the following vegetables.

To Stuff
Prepare one or more of the following:
1 small cabbage: cook it whole until the outer leaves have softened but the structure is still relatively firm. Cut off the top and, with a sharp knife, scoop out the central leaves and chop finely, add these to the filling.
large beetroot, cooked: peel, cut in half and scoop out most of the centre.
large onions: treat the same way as the cabbage.
marrow: cut in half lengthways, scoop out the centre, chop and use in the stuffing. You may like to bake this in the oven until it is slightly tender before stuffing.
butternut pumpkin: treat as for marrow.
leeks: cut off the green tops. Cut in half lengthways, remove central 'leaves' and use in the stuffing.

Assembly
Pile the stuffing into the vegetable shell(s) and place them in an oiled baking dish. Bake in a moderate oven for 30 minutes or until all ingredients are hot and cooked. Serve with a side salad and brown rice.

Variations
Include brown rice in the stuffing and reduce the amount of root vegetables. Stuff with Stir-fried Rice (p.131). Serve with a side salad to balance the rice.

Steamed Carrots with Dill

Ingredients
6 carrots, sliced on the diagonal   1 tablespoon fresh dill
1 teaspoon virgin olive oil

Method
Steam the carrots until just tender, drain and toss in the olive oil. Sprinkle the dill over the top and serve.

Variation
Week 5. Use almond oil instead of olive oil.

Leeks with Paprika

Ingredients

4 large fresh leeks, trimmed and
cut into lengths about 3" long
1 tablespoon virgin olive oil

3 large cloves garlic, finely
chopped
paprika

Method

Lightly steam the leeks until nearly tender, lay in a shallow oven dish.
Sauté the garlic in the olive oil until golden, pour over the leeks, sprinkle
with paprika and bake at 150°C for about 10 minutes.

Red Cabbage and Apple

Ingredients

$1/2$ red cabbage (depending on
size), shredded
olive oil

1–2 sweet apples, finely sliced
seasoning

Method

Stir fry the shredded cabbage, in sufficient olive oil to prevent it catch-
ing, until nearly cooked.
Add the sliced apple and continue to heat until both are well done.
Season and serve.

Variations

Add a finely sliced onion with the cabbage.
Use dark green cabbage instead (more nutritious than white cabbage)
and add a teaspoon of caraway seeds.

In The Future
Add a few sultanas at the start of cooking.

Vegetable Curry with Turmeric

Even if you don't like curry, don't skip this recipe, just leave out the
chilli powder and you will have a delicious vegetable dish with the benefit to your liver of the turmeric.

Ingredients

2 tablespoons olive oil
4 cloves garlic, chopped
1 cubic cm ginger, peeled and
chopped

2 large onions, finely chopped
1 heaped tablespoon turmeric
2 teaspoons coriander, ground
1 teaspoon cumin, ground

¹/₄ teaspoon each, ground
cardamom, mace, fenugreek
freshly ground black pepper
1–2 teaspoons hot chilli powder
(optional)
2 carrots, sliced
1 parsnip, sliced

¹/₄ small turnip, peeled and diced
¹/₄ small butternut pumpkin,
peeled and diced
stock or water
6 Brussels sprouts, halved
small head of broccoli, cut into
small pieces

Method

Heat the oil in a heavy-based saucepan or wok (wok is the easiest) and add the garlic, ginger and onions. Cook until the onions have begun to soften.

Add the spices and stir for five minutes. Add the carrots, parsnips, turnip and pumpkin and toss until coated with the spices. Add the stock or water and simmer until nearly cooked. Add the Brussels sprouts and broccoli and cook until just tender.

Serve with brown rice and accompanied by sliced banana and diced cucumber.

Variation

Week 5
Add 50 g of red lentils after adding the spices. Stir until they are coated with the spices, then add the vegetables and continue.

Week 3

Continue to select vegetable dishes from those above but you can now include potato, tomatoes, peppers and aubergines. You can also use this week's grains to make a variety of sauces to serve with them.

Beetroot Relish

You may find yourself looking for strong flavours to replace some of the processed sauces you used to eat. This one is tasty, good for your liver and permitted at this stage of the Liver Detox Plan.

Ingredients

100 g fresh horseradish, grated
(aids digestion and relieves
wind)

100 g raw beetroot, skinned and
grated (excellent for your liver)
1 small lemon, juiced

Method

Combine all ingredients, mix thoroughly, store in an airtight container and keep refrigerated. Serve a small amount to accompany a chicken dish.

Variation
In later weeks serve it with other meat dishes or with bean or other savoury dishes.

Vegetables with Herb Sauce
If you like a rich sauce on your vegetables, use the Herb Sauce below. You can use this in place of cheese sauces.
Pour it over freshly cooked vegetables before serving. Alternatively you can pour it over lightly cooked vegetables and bake in the oven for a short while.

Herb Sauce

Ingredients

250 ml rice milk
25 g barley flour
25 ml virgin olive oil

generous quantities of fresh herbs, e.g. parsley, chives, basil, dill weed, etc.

Method
Contrary to the elaborate instructions in many cookbooks, a sauce is very simple to make.
Make a paste in a small saucepan by slowly adding most of the milk to the flour and mixing thoroughly after each addition. Add the oil, bring up to boiling point, stirring continuously, and simmer until it has thickened and tastes cooked. Add the herbs, cook for another minute and serve.
Initially, it is best to add only a moderate amount of the 'milk' and add more as needed, when the mixture has thickened. In time you will know the quantities needed to achieve the consistency you like.

Variations
Week 3: You can use oat milk instead of rice milk.
Week 5: You can use wheat flour instead of barley flour.
In The Future: You can use cow's milk instead of rice or oat milk.

Green Beans with Tomato

Ingredients

500 g green beans *(this is an excellent recipe if the beans are slightly old and past their prime, but can also be made with more tender beans)*
5 medium sized onions, cut into rings

2 cloves garlic, finely chopped
1–2 tablespoons virgin olive oil
4 large tomatoes, sliced into rings
1 tablespoon fresh coriander or basil, chopped
1 tablespoon fresh parsley, preferably flat-leafed, chopped

Method
Use a skillet with a well-fitting lid.
Top, tail and string the beans. Cut on the diagonal into convenient lengths.
Sauté the onions and garlic in the olive oil until tender.
Lay the beans on the onions, then the slices of tomato rings. Sprinkle the herbs over the top, cover and simmer until the beans are tender, about 10–15 minutes depending on their size and age.

Variation
If you enjoy a Middle Eastern flavour, add some cumin seed or a small amount of ground cardamom.

Stuffed Aubergine

This is an excellent vegetable to stuff because of its rich flavour.

Ingredients

2 large aubergines, cut in half lengthways
3 tablespoons virgin olive oil
4 cloves garlic, crushed
4 large tomatoes, roughly chopped

2 tablespoons fresh basil, chopped
cooked brown rice
salt and freshly ground black pepper

Method
Bake the aubergine in a moderate oven until it begins to soften. Scoop out the centres, leaving just sufficient flesh attached to the skin to provide a viable shell. Meanwhile warm the oil, add the garlic and tomatoes, cook until soft, add the basil and the roughly chopped aubergine centre that you removed. Stir thoroughly.
Add sufficient rice to produce enough stuffing for the four aubergine halves. Season to taste and pile the mixture into the shells. Bake at 200°C until the aubergine shells are fully cooked.

Variation
Use a similar stuffing but place it into blanched sweet peppers from which you have removed the base and seeds.

In The Future
Cover with grated cheese and heat until it just starts to melt.

Greens with Chilli and Tomato

Any greens can be used for this dish, but ones with a strong flavour are best, such as mustard greens, escarole, collard greens, silver beetroot or spinach. If you like a milder flavour use sprouting broccoli that is mostly leaves with just a few 'sprouts'.

Ingredients
1 kg washed greens, chopped
3 large cloves garlic, finely
   chopped
2 medium onions, finely chopped
4 medium tomatoes, roughly
   chopped

2 tablespoons olive oil
1 red chilli, chopped, discard the
   seeds

Method
Chop the leaves and steam for about five minutes.
Sauté the onions, add the garlic, tomatoes and chilli.
Cook for two minutes, add the greens and heat through.

Variations

Week 5
Add 3 tablespoons of sunflower seeds.

In The Future
Add a few tablespoons of ricotta cheese or marscapone for the last minute of cooking and sprinkle with 2 tablespoonfuls of toasted sunflower seeds before serving.

Rice with Aubergine and Spices

Ingredients
1 clove garlic, chopped
1 large onion, chopped
2 large aubergines, chopped
2 green or red peppers, chopped
2 tablespoons olive oil
2 firm tomatoes, chopped
1 teaspoon turmeric powder (very
   good for your liver)

1 teaspoon ground coriander
1 teaspoon ground cumin
1 tablespoon each of chopped
   fresh basil and flat-leaved
   parsley
350 g cooked brown rice

Method
Sauté the garlic, onion, aubergines, peppers and spices in the olive oil until just softened, add the tomatoes and spices and cook until the tomatoes are soft. Add the herbs for the last minute of cooking.

Place the rice round the edge of a serving dish and pile the vegetable mixture in the centre.

Week 5

Continue to serve generous quantities of a wide variety of vegetables with each meal. Vegetables can now be served with herb sauces made with wheat flour, but again keep in mind that you want the vegetables themselves to be the major part of your diet.

Legumes
Legumes can be used as a side vegetable, but they can also make hearty meals in themselves. Use the following ideas either as a main dish or, by reducing the quantity, as a side vegetable to accompany fish, meat or poultry.

Kidney Bean Pilaf with Cumin

Ingredients

2 large onions, finely chopped
2 large cloves garlic, finely
   chopped
1 dessertspoon olive oil
2 teaspoons cumin seeds

150 g cooked red kidney beans
170 g cooked brown rice
a bunch of fresh chives, finely
   chopped

Method
Sauté the onions and garlic in olive oil until transparent, add the cumin seeds and stir. Add the rice and beans and heat until hot, stirring as needed to prevent them burning. Sprinkle with the chives and serve with vegetables.

Dahl with Turmeric

Not only does turmeric give this dish a delicious flavour and an interesting colour, but it is also very beneficial for the liver.

Ingredients

1 tablespoon olive oil
1 large onion, finely chopped
8 cloves garlic, finely chopped
1 heaped tablespoon turmeric

2 teaspoons coriander powder
200 g yellow or red lentils
water or vegetable stock
salt and black pepper to taste

Method
Heat the olive oil and sauté the onion, garlic and spices, stirring constantly to prevent burning. Add the lentils and continue to stir until coated with

the hot spices. Add the stock or water and simmer until the lentils form a smooth paste. Add more liquid as needed. Season to taste. This dish can be served as thick as mashed potato or nearly liquid in consistency.

Variation
Add more liquid and serve as a soup.

The Future

You can now add variety, especially in salads, by using some of the delicious nut and seed oils that are available. They include almond oil, walnut oil and apricot kernel oil. They are generally more expensive than olive oil but keep in mind that you are using them for their flavour as well as for their fat content. While you might think you can now use soy, corn or sunflower oil, it is better that you don't. They are much more processed than olive oil and present a greater challenge to your liver, so plan to continue using olive oil as you main oil long term.

Herb Sauce
You can now use cow's milk in the original sauce.

Cheese Sauce (Low Fat)
Make a cheese sauce as normal but use half the quantity of cheese. Season with English mustard and one of the vegetable stock powders you can buy from health food shops. They generally contain a variety of dried and powdered vegetables and herbs. Season with salt and white pepper. Adjust the quantities to suit your taste. These seasonings can augment the overall flavour without the need for so much cheese (or fat).

Braised Artichokes (2nd recipe)

This dish is repeated here, with variations, to remind you how good this vegetable is for your liver.

Ingredients

1 large onion, diced	100 ml dry white wine
3 cloves garlic, chopped	lemon juice
2 bay leaves	1 tablespoon chopped fresh herbs
3 tablespoons olive oil	200 ml stock
4 large artichokes	freshly ground black pepper to
1 tablespoon tarragon vinegar	taste

Method
Put the oil, onion, garlic and bay leaves in the base of a casserole dish just large enough to hold the artichokes and place in a preheated oven at

180°C for 10 minutes. Then place the artichokes in the dish, upright, baste with the olive oil and return to the oven for 10 minutes. Then add the vinegar and wine and return to the oven until the liquid has reduced by half (you will lose the alcohol but retain the flavours), after which time add the fresh herbs, lemon juice and stock, season, cover with the lid and allow to simmer for about an hour or until the artichokes are cooked and the liquid almost totally reduced.

Spicy Baked Beetroot

Ingredients

4 large beetroot
1 tablespoon almond oil
1/2 tablespoon balsamic vinegar

2 tablespoons sunflower seeds or
   chopped raw almonds

Method

Cut the leaves off the beetroot but take care not to damage the root or cut the skin. Boil or steam them until tender, peel and cut into chunks. Heat the almond oil in a heavy-based skillet or wok, add the beetroot and toss until thoroughly coated in the oil. Add the vinegar and seeds, toss again. Serve hot.

Variation

Beetroot is also delicious served hot with a white sauce, either plain or with added herbs.

Marrow in Paprika Sauce

This is a simple yet delicious way to serve marrow. It can also be done with other vegetables but works best with ones that are pale in colour and have a mild flavour. Other possibilities include cucumber or chokos if available.

Ingredients

1 large vegetable marrow or
   several courgettes
1 large teaspoon salt

1 dessertspoon olive oil
3 teaspoons sweet paprika
100–200 g plain yoghurt

Method

Slice and cut the marrow (or courgettes) into matchstick-shaped pieces. Sprinkle with the salt and set to one side for an hour or two, then drain off the liquid. Warm the olive oil in a heavy-based frying pan, add the paprika and stir, add the marrow strips and cook through, stirring occasionally and gently. When ready to serve, add the yoghurt. The amount will depend on how much sauce you want. Heat through and serve.

Variations
Add a few chopped mint leaves while cooking the marrow.
Sauté chopped onion or garlic and then add the marrow.

Main Dishes

Week 1

Grilled Fish

Ingredients

any fish of your choice, whole or as fillets or cutlets

olive oil
fresh herbs of your choice

Method
Lightly brush the fish with the oil and grill on both sides until cooked. Decorate with fresh herbs. Parsley is typical but a few sprigs of fresh coriander are a welcome variation.
Serve with fresh, lightly steamed vegetables (drizzled with a few drops of olive oil if you like) and brown rice.

Variation
Pan-fry the fish, use a low temperature and just a trace of olive oil.

Fish Stew

Ingredients

500 g root vegetables, include carrots, celeriac, turnip, swedes
250 g Brussels sprouts or other dark leaves
250 g leeks
500 ml Basic Stock (p.99)
500 g full bodied fish (cod or haddock are excellent)

3 tablespoons chopped fresh herbs of your choice (if you include fennel use only small amount as the flavour is strong)
salt to taste

Method
Prepare the vegetables, chop into small pieces and place in the stock in the bottom half of a double boiler. Put the fish, covered in the herbs, in the top. Season to taste. When all is cooked, combine, bring to a gentle simmer, decorate with fresh herbs and serve with brown rice.

Baked Fish

Ingredients

1 kg fish, filleted
olive oil
2 large onions, finely sliced
2 cloves garlic, finely chopped
4 sticks celery, cut into narrow
  lengths and steamed, in a
  minimum of water, until just
  softened

fresh dill weed
salt and pepper to taste

Method

Heat the olive oil in a heavy-based skillet, add the fish fillets and sear the outside. Set aside. Add the onions and garlic and sauté until transparent. Line the base of a casserole dish with the onions and garlic, and add the fish. Strain the celery and lay it over the fish. Sprinkle with the dill weed. Add sufficient liquid, either fish stock or the water in which the celery was steamed, to provide a depth of about 1 cm and keep the dish moist. Bake in a moderate oven for about 20 minutes. Add more liquid if necessary. Season to taste.

Baked Trout with Chervil

Ingredients

4 small trout
2 cloves garlic, crushed
5 tablespoons chopped chervil,
  plus sprigs to decorate
2 limes or half a small grapefruit,
  use finely grated rind (provided
  they are organically grown)
  and also the juice (if not
  organic use juice only)

6 shallots, cut into 2 cm lengths,
  the white part sliced lengthways as well

Method

Place the trout in a lightly oiled baking dish. Combine all other ingredients, and spread over the trout and set aside for an hour, turning them over two or three times. Bake at 150°C until the trout is cooked. Decorate with sprigs of chervil before serving.

Variation

Use whole fresh sardines instead of trout and marjoram instead of chervil.

Fish with Herb Stuffing

Ingredients

1 kg bream, cleaned, head
   removed
1 large onion, finely chopped
3 tablespoons olive oil
1 tablespoon fresh herbs, finely
   chopped

400 g cooked brown rice, very well
   cooked
salt and freshly ground black
   pepper

Method

Sauté the onion in olive oil. When golden and transparent, add the herbs, stir, add the rice and stir again thoroughly, season.

Stuff the bream with this mixture, lay them in an oven dish and brush with more olive oil. Add a small amount of water or fish stock (if you have it), just sufficient to prevent the dish drying out.

Bake in a moderate oven for about 30 minutes or until the fish is cooked. Serve with lightly steamed vegetables.

Prawn Pilau

Ingredients

3 tablespoons olive oil
3 cloves garlic, finely chopped
5 onions, diced
3 cardamom seeds
6 cloves
8 cm stick of cinnamon broken
   into 4 or 5 pieces
8 peppercorns

1 blade mace
350 g cooked brown rice,
   cooked in Basic Stock if
   available
1 cup cooked prawns
salt and freshly ground black-
   pepper

Method

Warm the oil in a heavy skillet, add the onions, garlic and spices, and cook until the onions are tender.

Add the rice and heat through, stirring sufficiently to prevent sticking or burning, then add the prawns and heat through, season to taste. Serve with a tossed salad.

Salmon Curry

Ingredients

2 tablespoons olive oil
6 cloves garlic, finely chopped
1 large onion, finely chopped
3 teaspoons ground coriander
2 teaspoons ground turmeric
1 teaspoon ground cumin
1/4 teaspoon ground ginger
1/2 teaspoon hot chilli powder

1/4 teaspoon ground nutmeg
1 tablespoon fresh lemon juice
salt and freshly ground black
   pepper
1lb fresh salmon steak or tinned
   salmon (fresh is best, but tinned
   can be used for convenience)

Method

Sauté the onions and garlic in the oil until tender, add the spices and cook for another minute. Drain the salmon, flake it into relatively large pieces, add to the spices and cook, stirring very gently to avoid breaking it up, until heated through. Add the liquid, if desired, and the lemon juice and season. Serve on brown rice, with, side dishes of sliced bananas and finely chopped fresh onions.

Burmese Fish Curry

Ingredients

1 kg fish
1 teaspoon turmeric
2 tablespoons lemon juice made
   up to a cup with water
2 tablespoons mustard oil
   (alternatively use mustard
   powder and olive oil, although
   the effect will not be quite the
   same)
3 onions, finely chopped

1 large head (lots of cloves!) of
   garlic, chopped
1 cubic cm fresh ginger root,
   finely chopped
2 green chillies (although these are
   technically peppers, which are
   not permitted until Week 3,
   chillies are acceptable here)
1 tablespoon fresh coriander
   leaves

Method

Rub the fish with some salt and then the turmeric, cut into strips and roll to season the cut sides. Allow to sit for an hour or two and then pour over the lemon juice and water and allow to soak, overnight if possible.
Heat the oil and sauté the onions, garlic and ginger. Add the whole chillies, fresh coriander leaves and the strips of fish and stir. Add sufficient water to just cover the fish and simmer until cooked.
Serve with brown rice and a dish of diced cucumber.

Stir-Fried Rice

Ingredients

2 tablespoons olive oil
1 large onion, chopped
3 large cloves garlic, chopped
the green tops of 3 shallots
1 carrot, grated
2 sticks celery, with leaves if
    tender, both chopped

fresh herbs of your choice
salt and freshly ground black-
    pepper
170 g cooked brown rice

Method

Warm the oil in a heavy-based skillet and sauté the onion and garlic. Add the shallot greens, carrot, celery and herbs. Add the cooked rice and herbs, mix thoroughly, season to taste. Serve with a side salad.

Variations

Add turmeric, paprika or other ground spices. Vary the vegetables used. Convert into a protein dish by adding cooked prawns or flaked fish.

Seafood Kebabs

Dill has a delicate flavour and doesn't mask the subtle flavours of the fish and prawns. If you use other herbs with a stronger flavour, reduce the quantity accordingly.

Ingredients

16 large prawns, peeled
200 g monkfish, cubed
200 g salmon, cubed
200 g cucumber, peeled, seeds
    removed and cubed

3 tablespoons citrus juice
    (grapefruit, lime, lemon or a
    combination)
2 tablespoons dill weed, chopped
1 clove garlic, crushed
2 tablespoons olive oil

Method

Thread alternating prawns, fish and cucumber onto skewers and lay on a flat platter. Combine the remaining ingredients, reserving some dill weed for decoration. Pour this over the kebabs and allow to marinade for one hour. Grill until the flesh is cooked, basting frequently with the marinade. Decorate with fresh dill and serve on a bed of brown rice, accompanied by a side salad.

Week 3

By now you should have become familiar with a wide range of fish and other seafood dishes. Now you may enjoy the addition of chicken, turkey and other birds to your repertoire, but do continue to eat fish several times a week.

You can, of course, simply roast or grill the chicken or other birds, but there are many other possibilities. Those below are just a tiny indication of what you can do.

You cannot use wheat flour yet, but barley flour makes a suitable substitute and you can make pastry, pancakes and a variety of interesting sauces with it. Include herbs and fruit *(see Chicken with Cranberry Sauce, also Substitutions)* to add interest.

Savoury Flan

This makes an excellent lunch for people on the move or at work. Using the Barley Pastry described below you can incorporate flans into your diet at this stage. Simply line a quiche dish with the pastry and fill it with any of the permitted foods. Use leftover chicken or fish and vegetables, add one or two beaten eggs, mix thoroughly and fill the flan shell. Bake at 200°C for about half an hour, until the pastry is cooked.

A simple trick is to cook, intentionally, an additional amount of dinner, and while it is cooking prepare the flan case. When your dinner is cooked, pile the extra food into the pastry case, pop it in the oven and let it cook while you relax for the evening. It will be ready in no time. Put it in the refrigerator and it will be ready to pop in your lunch bag in the morning. Make sure you also pack a finger salad to have with it.

Barley Pastry

You will be using barley flour for this pastry instead of the more usual wheat flour and a combination of oil, water and lecithin instead of having to work in butter and then add water. You will be delighted at how easy it is to make and use. Even when you can use wheat flour (Week 5), continue to make pastry using oil and lecithin in this way instead of butter.

Ingredients

25 ml olive oil	1 teaspoon lecithin granules
50 ml water	100 g barley flour

Method

Combine the water, olive oil and lecithin in a bottle. The amount needed will depend on the nature of the flour but it does no harm to have some of this mixture stored permanently in the fridge, ready for use. Place the barley flour in a bowl, shake the oil and water mixture, add some to the flour and mix thoroughly. If the mixture is too moist, add more flour. If it is too dry, add more of the liquid. Knead thoroughly and, if possible, let it 'rest' for half an hour. Roll out and use it to line a lightly oiled quiche dish.

Variations

From Week 5
You can use wheat flour if you prefer

In The Future
You can use pouring cream instead of the oil and water combination, however the latter is much healthier than cream and very tasty.

Chicken with Cranberry Sauce

Ingredients

2 chicken breasts
5 ml virgin olive oil
100 g cranberries
150 ml freshly squeezed orange
 juice

pinch nutmeg
salt and freshly ground black
 pepper to taste

Method

Warm the oil in a heavy-based skillet, add the chicken breasts and cook, turning occasionally, until tender. Add the cranberries, orange juice and nutmeg and seasonings and stir, scraping up any of the chicken juices or flesh caught on the pan. Serve the breasts and pour the sauce over them.

Grilled Orange Chicken

Ingredients

4 chicken breasts
1 orange (should be organically
 grown as you will be using the
 skin)

1 clove garlic, crushed
1 tablespoon chopped fresh basil
 (or other herbs)
freshly ground black pepper

Method

Make several slits in each chicken breast, using a very sharp knife. Using a fine grater, grate off the outer skin or zest of the orange, then juice the orange. Combine the orange zest and juice with the garlic, basil and pepper.

Lay the chicken breasts side by side, slit side up, on a baking tray and spread the mixture over them, working it into the slits. If you have time, allow this to sit for a while so the flavour can penetrate the flesh. Then grill the chicken until tender.

Serve the chicken, then add a tiny amount of hot liquid to the baking tray and use it to scoop up any of the flavouring that has stuck to the pan, pour over the chicken breasts.

Duck Delight

Ingredients

2 tablespoons olive oil
1 large onion, chopped
1 carrot, grated
1 beetroot, grated
2 tablespoons chopped fresh herbs
  (oregano and parsley make a
  good combination)

2 bay leaves
1 egg, beaten
85 g cooked brown rice
seasoning
1 duck

Method

Heat the olive oil, sauté the onion until transparent, add the carrot and beetroot, stir, then the herbs and cook for five minutes. Remove from the heat, allow to cool, add the beaten egg and then the rice. Season and use this mixture to stuff the duck.

Rub the duck with olive oil and (if liked) some crushed garlic or paprika. Bake in oven on 150°-180° for about three hours.

Turkey Breasts with Cherries and Lime

Ingredients

500 g turkey breast
1–2 tablespoons olive oil
juice of 2 limes

200 g fresh cherries, pitted
stock
salt and pepper

Method

Slice the turkey breasts so they are thin and sauté in olive oil over a low heat until they are tender. Add the lime juice, pitted cherries and sufficient stock to make gravy, heat through and season to taste.

Variations

Use other fruit instead of cherries.

In The Future

Use red wine instead of stock but add it to the cooked turkey and heat for a few minutes before adding the lime juice and cherries.

Week 5

You can now add wheat and corn, red meat, legumes, seeds and nuts to your diet. This will give you a wide range of options and you will be able to use many more recipes from your conventional recipe books.

Cassoulet

This is a simplified variation of the French version of our baked beans, tastier and more nutritious. In this version the typical sausages and fatty cuts of meat usually included have been omitted so it is kinder to your liver than the original.

Ingredients

300 g haricot beans
water or vegetable stock
500 g lean meat *(you can use beef, lamb, pork or even poultry – goose is traditional – either alone or in combination)*
2 tablespoons olive oil
2 cloves garlic, crushed
2 carrots, sliced

2 onions, sliced
4 tomatoes, chopped
2 bay leaves
$1/2$ teaspoon each of fresh thyme, marjoram and oregano, chopped
seasoning
fresh parsley to decorate

Method

If you have time, soak the beans in water overnight. Otherwise bring them to the boil, in water or vegetable stock, and allow to simmer for 10 minutes, then take off the heat.

Cut the meat(s) into small pieces, add to hot olive oil in a heavy-based skillet and heat until all the surfaces are sealed. Add the garlic and cook briefly. Place the meat in the bottom of a casserole dish. Add the vegetables and herbs to the pan, toss in the oil, scrape up the meat juices, adding some of the stock to accomplish this. Tip the mixture on top of the meat. Drain the beans and spread over the vegetables. Add sufficient stock to cover the beans.

Cook in the oven at 200°C for approximately 90 minutes, adding more stock if necessary. Season to taste and sprinkle over the chopped parsley.

Variation

In The Future
Use red wine to scrape up the meat juices.

The Future

You will now be able to choose main dishes from most of your recipe books, so there is little need to provide a lot of them here. Those below are just a few of hundreds of possibilities. The important thing to remember is to use only ingredients 'as they grow'. Use fresh tomatoes, for instance, rather than sauces in tubes with an ingredient list that leaves you confused. Add your own herbs and spices rather than the many commercial sauces with a variety of flavourings and colourings. Use meat as it comes from the bone rather than sausages or smoked or salted meats.

Tomato, Olive and Ricotta Sauce

This is an excellent accompaniment to grilled fish, poultry or meat dishes, or to put on vegetables.

Ingredients

2 cloves garlic, crushed
3 teaspoons sun-dried tomato
 paste
8 black olives, pitted and chopped
3 sprigs of coriander, basil or flat-
 leaved parsley

$1/2$ tablespoon chopped chives
freshly ground black pepper
100 ml ricotta cheese

Method
Combine all ingredients and adjust seasoning (and quantities) to taste.

Variation
Replace the ricotta with fromage frais.

'Tartare' Sauce

Greek yoghurt is used to lower the fat content of this tartare sauce.

Ingredients

5 tablespoons mayonnaise (either
 home made, or use a good-
 quality bought one)
5 tablespoons Greek yoghurt

1 bunch chives, chopped
1 bunch parsley, chopped
1 tablespoon chopped capers

Method
Combine all ingredients. Serve with fish.

Chicken with Nuts and Shallots

Ingredients

1 tablespoon wholemeal flour
1 teaspoon paprika
1/2 teaspoon cayenne pepper
2 chicken breasts, cut into strips
1 tablespoon virgin olive oil
1/2 tablespoon of butter
1 bunch shallots, remove green tops and cut into 2–3 cm lengths, on the diagonal, and chop the white stem
50 g nuts, finely ground (not peanuts)
50 ml white wine
250 ml vegetable stock
2 tablespoons plain (or Greek) yoghurt

Method

Mix the flour and spices. Add the pieces of chicken breast and mix until they are thoroughly coated and the flour has all been taken up. Warm the butter and oil in a heavy-based skillet or casserole dish. Add the chicken pieces, and white chopped shallots, toss and cook until fully seared. Add the wine and allow the alcohol to evaporate. Add the ground nuts and stock. Once simmering, turn the heat down and cook for an hour or until the chicken is very tender. Add the green tops of the shallots about 10 minutes before the end of the cooking time. Season, stir in the yoghurt and serve.

Variation

Use turmeric instead of paprika.

Beef Paprika

Ingredients

1 tablespoon paprika
1 teaspoon hot chilli powder
black pepper
1 tablespoon wholemeal flour
2 tablespoons olive oil
500 g lean beef, diced
150 ml full-bodied red wine
1 onion, diced
1 leek, thinly sliced
stock as needed
75 g quartered walnuts
2 tablespoons marscapone
chopped chives (or parsley) to decorate

Method

Combine the first three spices with the flour, add the meat and toss until it is well coated. Heat the olive oil in a skillet and add the coated meat. Continue to heat, tossing regularly to prevent burning, until the meat is just cooked. Add the wine and stir, allowing the alcohol to evaporate.

Add the onion and leek and continue cooking until they are soft, adding stock to provide liquid if needed. Add the nuts and stir in the marscapone. Serve decorated with chopped chives.

Spiced Lamb with Yoghurt

Ingredients

1 teaspoon ground coriander
4 cardamom seeds
1 teaspoon cumin seeds
1 teaspoon paprika
1 teaspoon chilli powder
1 teaspoon grated fresh ginger

4 cloves garlic, crushed
1 large onion, very thinly sliced
1 tablespoon fresh lemon juice
300 g plain yoghurt
500 g lean lamb

Method

Stir the spices, vegetables and lemon juice into the yoghurt and set aside. Trim all visible fat off the lamb, cut the meat into small cubes and add to the yoghurt mixture. Mix thoroughly and leave to marinate overnight.

Place the mixture in a wok or heavy-based skillet and cook, stirring occasionally, until the lamb is tender (the amount of time will depend on the size of the lamb cubes). If the mixture becomes too dry add some stock or water.

Variations

Replace the lamb with pork, beef or poultry.

Reduce the amount of yoghurt to 100 ml, stir the marinating meat more frequently, then cook by threading the lamb onto skewers and grilling it. Baste with the marinade from time to time.

Roast Lamb with Rosemary

This is an extremely simple way to produce a delightfully flavoured roast with a minimum of preparation time.

Ingredients

1 leg of lamb, boned
several large sprigs of rosemary

1 teaspoon French mustard
2 teaspoons olive oil

Method

Place the rosemary, intact, inside the lamb and close up. Combine the mustard and oil, spread this over the outer surface of the lamb. Roast the meat at 200°C for about 90 minutes (for a 1 kg leg) until well cooked, test near the end of this time.

Stuffed Pork Fillet

Ingredients
500 g pork fillets

1 tablespoon wholegrain mustard

4 cloves garlic, crushed

100 g mozzarella cheese

olive oil

Method
Make a slit down the centre of each fillet, not quite cutting it in half. Open it out and make two more parallel slits into the pork on each side of the central cut. This should leave you with a large surface area of pork exposed. Combine the mustard and garlic and spread over the pork. Lay thin strips of mozzarella cheese on top and close up the pork fillets. Secure with toothpicks. Wipe the outside of each fillet with olive oil and bake them in the oven at 180°C until the meat is tender.

Desserts

Week 1

During this week it is more important to have a salad starter with your main meal than a dessert. However if you do wish to have a dessert you should choose one of the fruit dishes (without rice) from Breakfast Dishes, Week 1.

Week 3

Your desserts must still be based on fruit, preferably fresh, so continue to select them dominantly from Breakfast Dishes, Week 1, but you can now use eggs to good effect, as in Apple Mousse *(see below)*. The following recipes will give you some additional choices and ideas. Keep in mind that spices and flavours such as nutmeg, cinnamon, mace, ginger and vanilla add the illusion of sweetness.

Using raw eggs whites means that for a short while your absorption of biotin (a vitamin) will be reduced. If you are fighting candida, biotin is important and you may want to avoid dishes that include raw egg whites.

Apple Mousse

Ingredients

6 sweet apples, peeled, cored and
   finely sliced
1/4 teaspoon cinnamon
1/2 teaspoon freshly ground nutmeg

1/4 teaspoon ground cloves
2 eggs, separated
500 ml rice milk
1 tablespoon agar

Method

Places the apples and spices in a saucepan with an absolute minimum of water, just enough to prevent sticking to the pan, and heat until they form a pulp. Allow to cool and stir in the beaten egg yolks. Mix the agar to a paste in a small amount of the rice milk, boil the rest of the rice milk and then add the agar paste and simmer for five minutes. Allow to cool slightly then add to the apple mixture, leave to cool completely.

Whip the egg whites until stiff, fold into the mixture, pile into individual serving glasses and allow to set.

Spicy Apple Sauce

Ingredients

1 teaspoon cinnamon
2 teaspoons nutmeg, freshly ground
1/2 teaspoon ground ginger

1/2 teaspoon mace
10 sweet apples, peeled, cored and
   chopped

Method

Combine the spices in the proportions shown. The amount of the final mixture you use will depend on the number of apples and on your own preference. If you have made too much, keep it in an airtight container for future use and remember it helps to mask the lack of sugar as these spices give an illusion of sweetness. Adjust spices to taste.

Lightly cook the apples with the spices in an absolute minimum of water, just sufficient to prevent sticking and burning, until tender. Use a double boiler if you have one. When soft, whip to a purée.

Variations

For a dessert, or as a sauce to serve with other desserts, use sweet apples but it can also be used as a sauce to serve with savoury dishes – simply choose tart apples, leave out the spices and add a dash of fresh lemon juice.

Use pears instead of apples.

Week 5
Fold in some sunflower seeds or crushed nuts.

Stuffed Oranges

Ingredients

4 oranges cut in half horizontally, juiced and then the flesh removed

120–200 g sweet potato, cooked and mashed (amount will depend on the size of the orange shells)

nutmeg, freshly ground, to taste
1 teaspoon vanilla essence
1 tablespoon poppy seeds
2 eggs, separated
8 mint leaves to decorate

Method

Combine the orange juice, sweet potato, nutmeg, vanilla essence and poppy seeds. Mix thoroughly and add the egg yolks. Whip the whites until stiff and firm, fold into the sweet potato mixture and pile this into the orange shells, decorate with mint leaves.

Baked Pears

Ingredients

4 ripe but firm pears (one per person)

4 tablespoons cooked buckwheat

freshly grated nutmeg

100 ml blackberry juice (*use frozen blackberries if the pure juice is not available, in which case use the berries for the stuffing and the liquid for basting*)

1 teaspoon olive oil
1x4" cinnamon stick, crumbled
4 cloves

Method

Cut the pears in half, scoop out the core and some of the flesh. Mash this flesh and mix with the buckwheat, nutmeg and moisten with sufficient blackberry juice to make a coherent stuffing. Fill the pears with the stuffing and place the two halves together again. Wipe the skins with olive oil, wedge the pears in a casserole dish so that they do not fall over, sprinkle the cinnamon over them, put a clove down the centre of each and add the rest of the blackberry juice to the dish. Bake in a moderate oven until well cooked, basting with the juice from time to time.

Pumpkin 'Pie'

This is a low-calorie version of a long-time favourite.

Ingredients

250 g butternut pumpkin, cooked and mashed
1 teaspoon ground cinnamon
1 teaspoon ground nutmeg
1/4 teaspoon ground ginger
rice milk
3 eggs, separated

Method

Place all ingredients except the egg whites in a blender and blend until smooth. The amount of rice milk should be sufficient to create a smooth cream without it being too runny. Whip the egg whites until stiff and fold into the mixture.

Serve in flat champagne glasses.

Variations

Line a flat baking dish with Barley Pastry, pile in the pumpkin mixture and bake at 150°C until cooked, about 45 minutes. Only have this dessert if your first course has been particularly light.

Week 5
You can now use wheat pastry. Make sure you use wholemeal flour.

Week 5

Desserts can now include nuts and seeds and this leads to some interesting dishes. Avoid using sugar but many of the dishes you are already preparing could be sweetened by adding fruit juice whenever a liquid is needed.

Apple Crumble

Ingredients

4 large, sweet, apples, cored and sliced
1/2 teaspoon mixed spice
100 g porridge oats
1 tablespoon tahini (sesame seed paste)
flaked almonds

Method

Lightly cook the apples and spices (in a minimum amount of water) until just tender. Put the mixture in an oven dish. Mix the oats and tahini thoroughly, then spread over the apple. Sprinkle with the flaked almonds. Bake in a moderate oven for about 40 minutes or until the oats are cooked.

Serve with Tahini Dressing *(see below)*.

Tahini Dressing

Ingredients

4 tablespoons tahini (sesame paste)

soy milk, rice milk or oat milk

Method

Slowly add the 'milk' to the tahini, stirring thoroughly. The mixture will gradually thicken, but then, as you add more of the liquid, it will quite rapidly get much thinner and reach a pouring consistency.

Variations

Use almond or cashew nut butter instead of tahini.
Soak a vanilla bean in the liquid before adding it to the tahini.

In The Future
Use cow's milk as the liquid if preferred.

Baked Pears with Almonds

Ingredients

4 large ripe pears, peeled, quartered and cored
50 g ground almonds
25 g flaked almonds
2 tablespoons almond oil

1 egg, lightly beaten
a few drops of almond essence
1 teaspoon nutmeg (these last two give the illusion of sweetness)

Method

Lay the pears in a lightly oiled casserole dish. Combine the other ingredients, sprinkle over the pears and bake in a moderate oven for 30 minutes or until well cooked. Serve with tahini dressing or coconut cream.

Variation

In The Future
Serve with plain yoghurt.

The Future

Because you can now add dairy products, a whole range of recipes that you will find in your own recipe books can be used. However do your best to omit sugar. Use a reduced amount of honey instead, or, better still, fruit juice and some of the spices you have already been using. To continue being kind to your liver, use ricotta cheese instead of cream cheeses (if called for) and plain yoghurt instead of cream. If making pastry, use the Barley Pastry recipe, using wholemeal wheat flour if you prefer, rather than a pastry made with white flour and butter.

Melon Basket

This is is a refreshing dish, when melons are in season (it should be excluded if you know you have candidiasis).

Ingredients
as many different melons as possible

Method
Cut the melons neatly in half.
Scoop the seeds and central or stringy pulp.
Using a melon scoop, remove the flesh from all of them and pile the melon balls into a dish.
Clean out the remaining pulp from the melon shells.
Pile the melon balls back into the shells and chill before serving.

Fresh Figs with Ricotta Cheese

Ingredients
The quantities for this dish can be left up to your personal preference.
fresh figs

ricotta cheese
liquid honey (optional)
pine kernels (or flaked almonds)

Method
Use a dark-coloured flat plate. Cover this with a layer of ricotta cheese. Slice the figs in half and place, face down, on the cheese until it is covered. Warm the honey slightly and drizzle it over the figs, add a small blob of ricotta to the centre and decorate with the pine kernels.

Dried Fruit with Vanilla

This is an excellent dessert for winter, when fresh fruit is not available.

Ingredients

dried fruit of your choice *(stone
    fruit such as apricots and
    pears work best, but use your
    imagination to create other
    combinations)*

1 vanilla pod

Method

Put the dried fruit and an equal volume of water (say 2 cups of each) in a casserole dish with the vanilla pod, cover and bake at 150°C for about 40 minutes. By the end the fruit should have absorbed nearly all the water. Add more if needed. The vanilla gives an illusion of sweetness and no sugar is needed.

Serve hot or cold with plain yoghurt or Tahini Dressing.

Exotic Bread Pudding

Dried fruit and orange juice provide the sweetness in this unusual school favourite, so the sugar is not missed.

Ingredients

150 g sultanas, currants and/or
    raisins
100 g unsulphured dried apricots
    and/or pears
rind and juice of 3 (organic)
    oranges
1 tablespoon rum

500 ml milk
1 vanilla bean
1 teaspoon grated nutmeg
4 eggs, lightly beaten
6–10 slices wholemeal bread
    (depending on thickness and
    preference)

Method

Soak the dried fruit in the orange juice and rum and allow to stand until all the fruit is fully softened. Use more liquid if necessary (if it is all absorbed), as some dried fruit is more moist than others. Meanwhile heat the milk, vanilla bean and nutmeg and keep warm for 30 minutes, then allow to cool. Remove the vanilla bean. Combine the milk and eggs and beat thoroughly.

Place alternating layers of the bread and fruit mixture in a lightly oiled casserole dish. Pour the egg and milk mixture over and set aside for 30 minutes to allow the custard to penetrate the bread.

Bake in a moderate oven for 30 minutes or until the custard has set.

Berry Cream

This dish can be made with fresh berries, however it is handy to have frozen ones in the deep freeze in case you have surprise guests. It is a light and refreshing dessert to have after a big meal.

Ingredients

frozen berries such a strawberries,   fromage frais or Greek yoghurt
   raspberries, blackberries, etc.

Method

Allow the fruit to thaw, strain off the juice and simmer to reduce the volume to a minimum.

Combine the fruit and fromage frais in the proportions that appeal to you. Add in the concentrated liquid and serve in elegant glasses.

Biscuits and Cakes

The Future

Biscuits and cakes have no part to play in the Liver Detox Plan since the emphasis has been on fruit and vegetables, even for snacks between meals. However now that you are planning The Future you may want to have some of these, so here is a possibility.

Nut Cake

Ingredients

125 g each of ground walnuts,   8 eggs yolks, lightly beaten
   almonds, cashews and hazelnuts   8 egg whites, beaten until stiff
   (500 g of nuts in total)   1 tablespoon honey

Method

Mix the egg yolks with the nuts and honey, the mixture will still be partially dry. Add a quarter of the beaten egg whites to the nut mixture and stir in (at this stage the mixture is so dry it is difficult to 'fold' them in). Add another quarter of the beaten egg whites, this time folding them in. Repeat until all the egg whites have been folded in, trying to keep as much air in the mixture as possible.

Place in a lightly buttered cake tin and bake at 160°C until a knife comes out clean and the cake is cooked.

Serve with plain yoghurt.

SECTION 2

If you are reading this book from cover to cover, you will already have read about the programme and are now going to learn more about why it is important. Alternatively, you may be starting here and then referring back to the programme described in Part 2.

Here we will look at where the liver is, what it does in relation to processing fats, proteins and carbohydrates, vitamins and minerals, and the role it plays in your immune and endocrine systems. We will then move on to the way your liver handles toxins and the effect of specific drugs, both social and medical. After that we cover some of the many things that can go wrong with your overall health when you liver starts to lose efficiency and underperform. Many hundreds of different symptoms and health problems can result from a faulty liver. Finally, you will learn some tests you can do to check out the state of your own liver.

If any part of what you are about to read seems too complicated, skip it. Some people want and need full explanations, others don't, while some need explanations just on particular topics. Other people just like to know that an explanation is available if they ever do want it. Keep in mind that you don't have to understand *all* the following details – or even understand *any* of them – for the Liver Detox Plan to work, but they may encourage you, should the temptations to break the diet ever pile up.

Part III

What your Liver Does

Anatomy

Your liver is one of the largest organs in your body, weighing in at around one and a half kilograms. It is roughly triangular in shape and lies on the right side of your abdomen, tucked up just beneath your diaphragm. Part of it is under your right rib cage, but a small part, the lower, central part, extends below your ribs and can be felt by hand pressure. Your gall bladder lies along this margin of the liver (later on you will learn how to find it). The liver is divided into two main lobes which are, in turn, divided into smaller lobes, called lobules. Between them are blood vessels and a fibrous web that supports the liver and helps to hold it in place.

A total of 1.7 litres of blood flows through your liver every minute. Put simply, it comes from two sources and serves two different purposes. Another organ that is similar in this regard is your heart. When your heart is doing its job, the blood enters from the rest of your body via a single large vein and flows through the heart's four chambers (and the lungs) as the heart acts on it in its role in the overall circulation system, sending it on its way, refreshed with oxygen, around your body. However your heart also has to look after itself and so some of the fresh blood doubles back and divides into thousands of tiny capillaries that feed all over the heart and supply it with oxygen and nutrients so it has the energy and nutrients it needs to do its job.

In a similar way blood flows through your liver for two reasons. First, blood comes to your liver from your heart via your hepatic artery. This divides and supplies the whole organ, feeding and nourishing your liver itself, providing oxygen and other nutrients, just as it does to your heart and all other organs and tissues in your body. When it has done that the blood collects up and leaves by the hepatic vein and goes back to your heart and lungs for reoxygenation.

The second type of blood arrives at your liver via the portal vein, and this is the blood on which your liver carries out so many of its roles, roles that are vital for the rest of your body. Picture your small intestine, a narrow tube about 2 cm in diameter (hence its name, 'small') and about 6 metres long. Now picture an interconnecting network of blood capillaries each contacting it for a small part of its length, so that, collectively they cover its entire length. The food you've eaten crosses the walls of your small intestine and enters the blood in these fine capillaries, all gradually joining up to form the portal vein, which carries this nutrient-rich blood to the liver. In this way the liver is intimately involved with receiving the products from your digestive system.

In addition to this relationship of your liver with your digestive tract there is another one and this involves the duct that carries bile from your liver into your duodenum (the beginning of the small intestine). This duct is actually made up of two ducts, the hepatic bile duct and the cystic duct. During a meal the hepatic duct delivers bile directly from the liver into the duodenum to aid fat digestion (this duct becomes particularly important if you have your gall bladder removed). When there is no food in your digestive tract, this duct diverts the bile to your gall bladder, where it is stored for later use. Then when bile is once again needed your gall bladder contracts and squirts the bile along the cystic duct which connects up with the hepatic duct and the combination, now called the common bile duct, delivers bile to your duodenum.

You will sometimes hear the liver referred to as a gland as well as an organ. A gland is a part of your body that produces and secretes a substance that goes to another part of the body and affects its function. Since your liver makes and secretes bile that is stored in your gall bladder and then transported to your duodenum, where it performs its functions, it is considered to be an exocrine gland, since its impact, in this function, is *outside* the body. It is *outside* your body in the sense that it is not an intimate part of it, instead it is a cavity within the overall space of your body, just as your mouth is. The intestines, in other words, are connected to the outside air. An endocrine gland (as opposed to an exocrine one) affects other organs or tissues inside the body, such as the kidneys, heart or lungs.

Digestion

That, then, is a brief description of your liver. It is now time to explore what it does in relation to digestion and to do this we need to know a little more about the various types of food we eat. We will first consider the fats, then we'll consider the other foods, the protein and carbohydrates.

To be specific, the term 'digestion' actually covers three steps: ingestion, digestion and absorption. Ingestion is the putting of food in your mouth, digestion is the combination of processes that happen within the digestive tract, absorption is the transfer of digested food particles across the walls of the small intestine and into the bloodstream. This is followed by metabolism, the processes that occur as the various cells and body fluids process what has been absorbed. We're now going to look at the overall role of the liver in digestion and metabolism.

Fats

The liver has a huge role to play in the metabolism of fats, just because they are not water soluble. How it is accomplished depends on the type of fat in question, so let's take a look at that first.

There are two major groups of fats or oils. First there are the so-called 'mineral oils'. These are the substances obtained from oil wells and their structure is so different from the oils you consume from your diet or make within your body that you cannot even metabolise them. If, for instance, you eat a mineral oil, such as liquid paraffin, it is not digested or absorbed, but simply goes straight through the digestive tract, acting as a laxative. It can even do harm, as it may dissolve some of the fat-soluble vitamins from your diet, taking them out with it.

The second group of fats are the fats, or lipids, found in plants, animals and human beings. The term 'lipids' covers both fats (solid) and oils (liquid). For this section we will refer to them in this way most of the time, though when we revert to talking about foods it is often easier to go back to referring to them by their common name, fats.

Although lipids are spoken of as if they constitute a coherent group of compounds, they are actually very different. What they *do* have in common is the fact that they feel 'oily' and they do not dissolve in water.

You may have come across terms such as 'saturated' and 'unsaturated' fats, 'triglycerides' and 'cholesterol', even perhaps 'trans fatty acids', yet may not know precisely what these are. Because lipids are so important, and because your liver is the main organ that deals with them, it is helpful to develop some understanding of them – although if you don't want a great deal of detail you can, of course, skip this section.

Table 6: **The types of fats and their sub-groupings**

ORGANIC LIPIDS

1 FATTY ACIDS – long carbon chains

2 TRIGLYCERIDES – composed of fatty acids and glycerol

3 WAXES – composed of fatty acids and different alcohols

4 PHOSPHOLIPIDS – lipids that contain a phosphate group
   a) **Lecithins** – similar to triglycerides but include choline, serine, ethanolamine and inositol.

5 MISCELLANEOUS SPECIALISED LIPIDS

6 STEROIDS – composed based on variations of the steroid nucleus
   a) **Cholesterol**
   b) **Adrenal cortex hormones**
       (i)   Cortisone
      (ii)   Cortisol
     (iii)   Corticosterone
      (iv)   Hydrocorticosterone
       (v)   Aldosterone
      (vi)   Female hormones
             (a) Oestrogen
             (b) Estrone
             (c) Estradiol
             (d) Progesterone
             (e) Pregnanediol
     (vii)   Male hormones
             (a) Testosterone
             (b) Androsterone

7 FAT-SOLUBLE VITAMINS
   a) Vitamin A
   b) Vitamin D2 and D3
   c) Vitamin E

MINERAL OILS

Parrafin

Hexane

Benzene

Other petroleum derivatives

Types of Fat

Fatty Acids

The first group of lipids consists of fatty acids. These are the simplest components of the lipid group. They do not occur on their own, to any significant extent, either in food or in your body, but they are the basic component of many lipids, particularly of the triglycerides, and they are released when these are broken down during digestion.

Individual fatty acids occur in a wide range of foods and most fats contain a variety of different fatty acids. Some of these are essential for health.

Table 7: **Examples of individual fatty acids**

Name	No of C atoms	Saturation	Occurrences (examples only)
Butyric acid	4	saturated	butter
Caproic acid	6	saturated	butter
Caprylic acid	8	saturated	coconut oil
Capric acid	10	saturated	palm kernel oil
Lauric acid	12	saturated	coconut oil
Myristric acid	14	saturated	nutmeg oil
Palmitic acid	16	saturated	most animal and plant lipids
Palmitoleic acid	16	mono-unsaturated	butter
Stearic acid	18	saturated	most animal and plant lipids
Oleic acid	18	mono-unsaturated	olive oil
Linoleic acid	18	di-unsaturated	linseed, evening primrose
Linolenic acid	18	tri-unsaturated	linseed, evening primrose
Arachidic acid	20	saturated	peanut oil
Arachidonic acid	20	tetra-unsaturated	lecithin

The above examples are only that, examples. The individual fatty acids occur in a wide range of foods, especially those fatty acids with sixteen or eighteen carbon atoms. As you look at the table you may be in for some surprises. It may, for instance, surprise you to see that palmitoleic acid, an unsaturated fatty acid, occurs in butter, or that vegetable oils, such as palm kernel oil, contains capric acid, a saturated fatty acid. It is true that butter is generally considered to be a saturated fat and vegetable oils to be unsaturated, but most fats contain a variety of different fatty acids, some of them saturated, some of them unsaturated. In the case of butter, most of them are saturated. In vegetable oils a higher proportion of the fatty acids are unsaturated, but there are also some saturated ones.

So, it is now time to learn what saturated really means. **Saturated fatty acids** are ones in which every carbon atom in the chain is saturated with hydrogen.

Essential Fatty Acids

Your body uses most fatty acids for the production of energy, but there are three noteworthy fatty acids. They were, at one time, called the three 'essential fatty acids'. When a nutrient is called 'essential' it means that it is vital for life and that without an appropriate supply of it in your diet you die, rapidly; in contrast, 'important' nutrients are ones that are protective and help to prevent health problems developing in the longer term.

The three fatty acids are called linoleic acid (LA), linolenic acid, properly called alpha-linolenic acid (ALA) and arachidonic acid (AA), and they are all polyunsaturated. Although it may be slightly confusing, it is worth mentioning that there is a second form of linolenic acid called gamma-linolenic acid (GLA). This is formed from linoleic acid and should not be confused with ALA. You will often find the term GLA on some supplements of the essential fatty acids, including supplements with evening primrose oil which contains some.

Linoleic acid comes mainly, but not exclusively, from seeds and hence from vegetable oils. Linolenic acid comes mainly from fish but is also found in a few plant seed oils such as evening primrose oil, borage oil and linseed oil. Arachidonic acid comes mainly from animal sources but is also found in vegetable oils. Linoleic acid is essential in the diet, linolenic acid is probably essential, it is certainly very important and protective. Arachidonic acid is not essential, as anything it can do, we now know, linoleic acid can also do. In fact you may eat too much of it, in which case you can get some unwanted symptoms such as inflammatory reactions and an increased tendency of your blood to clot (useful when you need it, but a danger at other times). All these fatty acids perform several roles – they are part of the structure of cell walls, they are components of lecithin, an extremely valuable nutrient for your liver, and they are converted into groups of compounds called the prostaglandins.

Prostaglandins

Prostaglandins are extremely important compounds, involved in the fine tuning of the way your individual cells and tissues function. In a sense, you can consider them to be mini hormones. Hormones are made in glands, such as your adrenal glands, and then travel through your blood to the target tissues, such as your heart and muscles, where they exert their reaction, such as increasing your heart rate and giving you the energy to run or fight. Hormones can have a lifetime of many minutes; you have doubtless felt the prolonged beating of your heart after a fright and a rush of adrenaline.

Prostaglandins, on the other hand, are made and used on the spot. For instance when a blood cell hits the wall of the artery (something that is happening billions of times a second) the cell pumps out the appropriate prostaglandin (one of the PG3 series, we will learn about in a minute), one that gives the instruction 'Don't clot' and the blood flows on its way. On the other hand, if you get a pinprick, the affected cell pumps out a different prostaglandin (one of the PG2 group), one that gives the opposite instruction and causes your blood to form a clot.

This is not the place to go into a detailed discussion of prostaglandins, however a few comments are in order. Each series consists of a large number of compounds, all with different jobs to do, and we certainly won't be going into them all. In general, however, the PG1 series is mildly anti-inflammatory and anti-thrombotic (reduces the tendency of the blood to clot). The PG2 series is highly inflammatory and includes, for instance, a group of compounds called leukotrienes that are tens, even hundreds of times more inflammatory than histamine, and histamine can cause some pretty nasty allergic (and inflammatory) reactions. It also encourages blood to clot, which is great when you have a cut but undesirable if your blood shows a tendency to form thrombi that can slow it down or block its flow round your circulatory system and thus lead to circulatory and heart problems.

Trans Fatty Acids

The more unsaturated a fatty acid is, the lower is its melting point and it tends to be liquid rather than solid at room temperature. This means that to make margarine (solid) from vegetable oils (liquid) some of the fatty acids have to be 'hydrogenated' (by the addition of hydrogen to some of the sites from which it was missing). However, in doing this not only is hydrogen added to some of the double bonds, but others, that remain as double bonds, are changed in their shape. In some cases, the gaps where the hydrogen has been removed from each end of a double bond are on the same side of the chain. These are called cis (same) double bonds, hence 'cis fatty acids'; these are the good guys and are rarely spoken of. However, in other cases the double bonds that do remain can be changed so the gaps are on opposite sides of the chain to each other. They are then called trans (opposite) double bonds, hence 'trans fatty acids'.

These trans fatty acids are the bad guys – they are abnormal fatty acids, they do not occur naturally and they can block a number of normal metabolic processes. They constitute one of the problems of eating hydrogenated margarine or any fats that have been hydrogenated; this includes fats that have been heated to a high temperature such as occurs in deep-fat frying.

We will be talking more about them shortly.

Triglycerides

Lipids, as already mentioned, do not occur in food in the form of free fatty acids. Instead most of the lipids you eat come in the form of a combination of three fatty acids attached to glycerol. These larger molecules are called triglycerides and triglycerides make up the majority of the fats in meat and other flesh foods, butter, vegetable oils, avocados, nuts and other high-fat foods.

Rancid Fats

One of the problems that can occur in the fats you eat is rancidity. You've almost certainly seen the way the outer layer of butter becomes a darker colour than the central part. The outer layer has become rancid, and rancid fats should not be eaten.

There are two ways fats can go rancid: hydrolysis and oxidation. Hydrolysis gives food its unpleasant taste and oxidation occurs to unsaturated fats and can lead to the formation of highly toxic compounds, some of which are carcinogens.

Phospholipids

The phospholipids are a large groups of compounds and many of them need not concern us here, however one group is particularly important and that is the phosphatides.

Phosphatides

Phosphatides are similar to triglycerides, but contain only two fatty acids, selected from a group of six, namely linoleic, linolenic, arachidonic, palmitic, stearic and oleic acids. In place of the third fatty acid there is a phosphate group (hence their name) and one other group, as indicated by the name of the particular phosphatide. The group attached to the phosphate can be either choline, inositol, serine or ethanolamine. You may have heard of choline, inositol or serine, as they occur in many vitamin supplements, particularly in multi-vitamins and in B complexes.

When either choline or inositol is included, the compound is called lecithin which, as already mentioned, is essential for the health of your liver. If you want to, or have been recommended to, add choline or inositol to your list of supplements, it is better to take them as lecithin than on their own. This way they are protected within the lecithin molecule and so avoid being broken down or damaged within the digestive tract.

Cholesterol and Other Steroids

This is a large group of compounds, all based on the steroid nucleus and commonly derived from cholesterol. Cholesterol is important both in itself and also because it helps in many important functions in the body:

- under the skin with the action of light it is converted into vitamin D
- in the liver it is essential for the formation of bile and hence for fat digestion
- in the adrenal glands it is converted into cortisone, cortisol, corticosterone, aldosterone and other vital compounds
- in the ovaries and adrenal glands it is converted into the female sex hormones such as oestrogen and progesterone
- in the testes and adrenal glands it is converted into the male sex hormones such as testosterone and androsterone
- cholesterol itself is a component of cell membranes and of the brain and nervous system

The Fat-Soluble Vitamins

The fat-soluble vitamins are vitamins A, D, E and K:

- Vitamin A is half the beta-carotene molecule. It is an important antioxidant, needed by the skin and mucous membranes, and essential for sight.
- Natural vitamin D (D3), is made from cholesterol, while the synthetic form (D2) is made from ergosterol, a plant steroid. It is needed for the absorption of calcium.
- Vitamin E is a group of compounds called tocopherols (alpha-, beta-, gamma-, delta-, eta- and zeta-tocopherol). They exist in d- and l- forms, which are mirror images of each other. The d- form occurs naturally and is important for health. Synthetic forms generally contain both d- and l-tocopherols, but the l- form is of little use and may cause harm. Vitamin E is an antioxidant and helps protect your heart and improve healing.

- Vitamin K is essential for blood clotting. Much of what you get is made by the bacteria in your gut, a reaction that is greatly reduced when you take antibiotics that kill off these bacteria.

Fat Digestion

Now you know something of the different types of fats it is important to see what your liver has to do to digest them.

The lipids you ingest first melt in the warm environment of your mouth and stomach, and then form globules. The churning action of the stomach breaks down these globules into tiny droplets and these move on into the duodenum, where they can be acted on by lipases or lipid-splitting enzymes. However these enzymes can only act on the surface of each globule or droplet. One large globule presents a very much smaller surface area than is presented by the thousands or even millions of separate tiny droplets into which it can form. Since, during digestion, the lipids keep moving along the intestines, there is a finite length of time during which the enzymes can act on and digest them, and by the time the enzymes have worked even a small part of the way through a large globule it would be on its way out of your body, in the stool. It is therefore essential that the lipid is held in the form of millions of tiny droplets so that digestion can occur rapidly, and be complete before the food has left your small intestine. Keeping the lipid in the form of these tiny droplets is where the liver is involved.

Let's digress a minute and think about making salad dressing. Normally, when you shake up a mixture of oil and water, such as oil and vinegar when making a salad dressing, you first achieve a fine mixture of the two. Then, on standing, all the tiny lipid droplets come together and float on top, and all the water (or vinegar) droplets come together and remain on the bottom. If you want to prevent this separation happening you need an emulsifying agent. This is a substance with a dual characteristic, one end of the molecule is lipid soluble and the other end is water soluble. The lipid-soluble end dissolves in a tiny droplet of lipid and the water-soluble end in a droplet of water. Think of the emulsifying agent as a dumbbell, with a droplet of lipid at one end and water at the other. Once that structure is established, no matter how hard all the lipid droplets try to come together, they can't. Possibly five or six droplets can come together, then their associated water molecules get in the way. As a result of this emulsifying action the tiny droplets are maintained and a large surface area of lipid is presented to the lipases (fat-splitting enzymes) and digestion occurs smoothly and in the right part of the digestive tract. What is the emulsifying agent? It is bile, a complex substance that contains bile salts, bile acids, cholesterol and lecithin and is produced by the liver, stored in the gall bladder and squirted down the common bile duct into the duodenum every time you eat food that contains fat.

Bile performs at least four functions. It emulsifies the fat that has entered the duodenum as part of the diet; this is done by the bile acids in combination with lecithin. It stimulates the release of lipases, the enzymes needed for the breakdown of lipids, from the pancreas. It combines with the lipids to form micelles, or water-soluble complexes from which the lipid or fat part can be easily absorbed further down in the small intestine. Finally, it stimulates peristaltic action, the muscular movements of the walls of the digestive tract, that propel the foods along; by doing this it helps to prevent stasis and constipation

The Gall Bladder

It is time now to consider your gall bladder in more detail. It is an elongated pear-shaped sac, about 10 cm long and two to three cm wide, lying below the liver and attached to it. As you now know, bile that has been made in the liver to the gall bladder, where it is concentrated and stored. Bile, as it leaves the liver, is 97 per cent water. In the gall bladder it is concentrated and is reduced to 89 per cent water. This concentration means it takes up less space, however it also increases the risk of some of the solids precipitating and forming stones, known as 'gallstones'.

Following appropriate stimulation, such as the presence of fat in the digestive tract, your gall bladder contracts, thus squirting bile down another duct, the cystic duct, then into the common bile duct, and finally into the duodenum where, as we have already seen, it is essential for normal fat digestion. Other substances can also trigger the contraction of the gall bladder, and, collectively, they are called cholagogues. You will, for instance, find a number of herbs referred to as cholagogues, and these are the ones that stimulate the function of the gall bladder. Strictly speaking, substances, including herbs, that stimulate the flow of bile are called choleretics, but in fact, the term 'cholagogue' is often used to cover both actions.

Bile Production

On average, a healthy liver produces and secretes about half a litre of bile a day. The main components of bile are bile salts, bile pigments, cholesterol, bile acids and lecithin *(see Table 8)*, dissolved in an alkaline solution, somewhat similar to the digestive juice that flows from the pancreas.

Table 8: **The composition of bile**

		Without water
Water	97%	
Bile salts	0.7%	35%
Inorganic salts	0.7%	35%
Bile pigments	0.2%	10%
Fatty acids	0.15%	7%
Lecithin	0.1%	5%
Fat	0.1%	5%
Cholesterol	0.06%	3%

Once this bile has played its role in lipid digestion within the small intestine one of two things can happen. Some of it remains in the small intestine, moves on to the colon or large intestine and then leaves the body as part of the stool. The bile pigments, for instance, are what gives your stool its colour, without them it would be a pale grey or white. However most of the bile solution is reabsorbed from the end of your small intestine, just before it joins the colon, and is returned, via the blood, to your liver. For instance 95 per cent of the bile salts are reabsorbed. This closed loop is known as the 'enterohepatic circulation' and the bile circulates continuously in this way, approximately twice for each meal or six to eight times a day. This is particularly important, as you will see later, when we come to discuss how to get rid of excessive amounts of cholesterol if your blood level is too high.

Cholesterol

It's time now to consider the cholesterol in bile. Although cholesterol itself forms only a small part of the bile, the bile salts (forming 35 per cent) are also based on cholesterol.

In spite of its bad reputation, cholesterol is an extremely valuable substance, performing many different essential actions in the body and being the starting-point for a variety of essential compounds. So important is it that if you don't eat a sufficient quantity of cholesterol you manufacture it yourself to make good the shortfall. In fact the average consumption of cholesterol from dietary sources is only about 300 to 500 mg/day, mainly from eggs, meat and dairy products, whereas the daily requirement is 1,100 mg, which means that over half the cholesterol you need, every single day, has to be synthesised within your body. This is done either in the cells lining the small intestine or in the liver. The amount synthesised by the small intestines increases with the amount of fat you eat as it is needed to transport the fat to the liver. Your liver, provided it is healthy, only produces cholesterol if your body needs an additional amount for the different roles it performs.

What does all this mean? For one thing, it means that that there is little point in trying to reduce your blood cholesterol level by eating less cholesterol (unless you are eating more than 1,100 mg a day), since then your liver will simply make more. There is some point in reducing your total fat intake, as less cholesterol will then be synthesised by the cells lining your small intestine and this leaves the job of fine-tuning the amount that is produced to the liver. It also leads to less fat for your liver to deal with. Your liver, provided it is healthy, then responds to high levels of cholesterol in the blood by synthesising less.

Problems with cholesterol consumption do start if you eat oxidised cholesterol. In practical terms, this means that you should eat soft cooked eggs rather than hard cooked ones, particularly if the shell is removed prior to cooking. Eat soft-boiled eggs, soft scrambled eggs or runny omelettes rather than their overcooked counterparts.

A much richer source of cholesterol is brains. These contain about four times the amount of cholesterol that is found in the same weight of eggs. This highlights the large need for cholesterol by the brain to do its job. Another factor in favour of eggs is that they contain a high concentration of many of the other nutrients you need, including lecithin which helps you to metabolise the cholesterol safely. In fact, if you got 10 per cent of your calories from eggs, you would get a lot more than 10 per cent of a large number of the essential vitamins and minerals you need, sometimes as high as 50 per cent or more (this makes sense, as the chicken would hardly go to the trouble of laying a bulky egg full of non-nutritive substances, the egg is a compact package of all that is needed for a developing life).

Some of my patients express concern about the 'cholesterol' in crayfish and prawns. In fact, though related, this is a slightly different compound and is only poorly absorbed, so it need not concern you, and the low fat content of this form of protein is an advantage.

Bile Acids

There are four bile acids, called cholic acid, chenodeoxycholic acid, deoxycholic acid and lithocholic acid. They are all made from cholesterol via cholic acid. Cholic acid and chenodeoxycholic acid are the main two. The other two are also formed in the colon by the action of bacteria on the first two.

Bile Salts

The bile salts are the sodium or potassium salts of the bile acids in combination with one of two amino acids, either glycine or taurine, the latter being made from another amino acid, cysteine, which contains sulphur.

As a result the bile salts are known as either 'glycocholic acid' or 'taurocholic acid'.

Glycine is a relatively common amino acid and can be made in the body. Taurine deserves a further discussion and we will talk more about it later, particularly when considering what to do for an unhealthy liver. We will also be talking about cysteine in this regard. You will find that these two amino acids, cysteine and taurine are recommended as supplements to take if your liver and gall bladder are sluggish.

Bile Pigments

There are two main pigments in bile, called biliverdin and bilirubin, which give the bile its golden-yellow shade and also colour the stool. Bilirubin is formed by the breakdown of haemoglobin, the red colouring material in red blood cells. This free bilirubin travels through the blood attached to the protein albumin. Further reactions occur in the liver to produce the final bile pigments. One of these reactions will be talked about later, in regard to the way the liver deals with toxins, so it is worth describing it here.

One of the steps in this process is the addition of a substance called glucuronic acid to the bilirubin. The process is called glucuronidation and the result is called a glucuronide. Thus the bile pigments are actually glucuronides of bilirubin. This is important as it is a way the body deals with a number of unwanted or toxic compounds including old and used cholesterol and drugs such as anticonvulsants, antihistamines and barbiturates. The formation of these bilirubin glucuronides is an important step in the liver's work of packaging unwanted drugs and other toxins and eliminating them via the bile duct, into the intestine and out in the stool.

Lecithin

Lecithin is another component of bile, one that is enormously valuable for your liver:

- It is an emulsifying agent.
- It is an essential component of bile and helps to prevent stones forming and precipitating out, thus helping to prevent gallstones.
- It is essential for the liver itself.
- It is an essential component of lipoproteins *(see below)* and thus for the safe transport of lipids through the bloodstream.
- It is a source of choline and inositol, which also play vital roles both in the liver and elsewhere. Choline, for instance, is essential (as acetyl choline) for your nerves to be able to pass messages from one to another, while inositol is important in the brain and nerve sheaths.

Fat Absorption and Transport

We have now covered the nature of fats, their digestion and the role of your gall bladder and the bile it supplies. The next step is the absorption of these fats, once they have been broken down into some of their components.

Once these components have been released and absorbed they coalesce back into relatively large fat droplets and these have to be packaged in such a way that they can be carried through the blood. To achieve this they are combined, once they have crossed the intestinal wall, with cholesterol (either from the diet or manufactured on the spot), lecithin and protein to form complexes called 'chylomicrons' and 'lipoproteins'.

There are three main lipoproteins called VLDLs (Very Low Density Lipoproteins), LDLs (Low Density Lipoproteins) and HDLs (High Density Lipoproteins) and their composition is shown in the chart below. Chylomicrons and VLDLs are formed in the small intestinal walls and these then travel through your blood, finally reaching the liver. If you have eaten a high-fat meal this can put a considerable burden on the bloodstream, in fact, after a high-fat meal your blood becomes so full of them it can even look white and cloudy as a result. When you look at the blood under the microscope you can see a blizzard of thousands of droplets of fat filling the spaces between the cells. A look at that alone has often been sufficient to stop many of my patients eating a high-fat meal ever again.

Table 9: **The composition of chylomicrons and lipoproteins**

	Size (nm)	Protein %	Cholesterol %	Triglycerides %	Lecithin %
Chylomicrons	75–100	2	5	90	3
VLDLs	30–80	10	12	60	18
LDLs	20	25	50	10	15
HDLs	7–10	50	20	5	25

Once these fats have started on their route through the blood the next steps are relatively complicated, but the following simplified picture will help you to understand what happens.

As you can see from the table above, the chylomicrons are particularly rich in triglycerides and so they travel round your body delivering triglycerides to the various tissues that need them for the production of energy. If energy is not required, the remainder of the triglycerides are delivered to your adipose tissues (your spare tyres and the bulges you don't want) and stored as fat until such time as they may be needed. In addition, some of your tissues will want the essential fatty acids, linoleic acid and linolenic acid that are in these triglycerides.

Once stripped of most of their triglycerides, the chylomicron remnants go to the liver, where they are repackaged into VLDLs, using any fat that is in the liver and also into HDLs.

The VLDLs, from both the small intestine and the liver, also deliver their triglycerides. As they do so, they become less dense and relatively more rich in the other components, the cholesterol and protein. They thus gradually turn into LDLs, which travel through the bloodstream and deliver cholesterol to the tissues that need it. As already mentioned, cholesterol has many uses and is needed in many different parts of your body.

It is now the turn of the high-density lipoproteins, the HDLs. These travel through the bloodstream, passing one type of tissue after another and picking up the 'spent' cholesterol. They then take it to the liver, where it can be made into bile acids and salts and secreted as bile. Part of this cholesterol (something like 10 per cent) is then lost in the stool, and part of it (around 90 per cent or more) is reabsorbed and transported back to the liver for recycling.

There is one very important aspect of cholesterol metabolism. Whereas most other large molecules can be broken down in the body into carbon dioxide and water, with energy being released in the process, there is no mechanism for breaking down any unwanted cholesterol. Thus the *only* way you can get rid of any excess of cholesterol from your body is via the stool, in the bile.

If this whole sequence of reactions happens perfectly this will contribute to your good health. However there are many ways this sequence of events can go wrong. Trans fatty acids can hinder the formation of HDLs or the conversion of LDLs to HDLs. If this happens there can be a back-up of LDLs in the blood and so your blood cholesterol level will rise. This is dangerous and unhealthy. However the answer is not to reduce your intake of cholesterol – that was not the cause of the problem – but to stop consuming hydrogenated fats or fats that have been heated to a high temperature.

There is, happily, a nutrient that works in the opposite direction. Vitamin C encourages the production of HDLs and so helps to maintain a low blood cholesterol level. It benefits in other ways, too, as it helps to keep the cholesterol in solution and reduce its uptake by any atheromas that may be forming along the artery walls.

It is also important that your liver is healthy enough to do its job of getting rid of the chylomicron remnants and the fats released from them and of making the HDLs. In these ways you can help to reduce your risk of having a heart attack.

Fat Metabolism

With the exception of cholesterol, most fats, if not stored in adipose tissues, are used for the production of energy. The triglycerides are broken down into fatty acids. These then get split into segments that are two carbon atoms long, called acetyl groups, that are further broken down in the Krebs cycle. This step is called 'ketogenesis', the formation of ketones. The reason it is important to mention this here is that if you eat a large amount of fat and very little carbo- hydrate this Krebs cycle stops running and you are left with the ketones. It's like standing beside a merry-go-round but not being able to get onto the animals for the ride. This is important, as many diabetics know.

Once the triglycerides are in the bloodstream (whether they have come from the diet or been released from adipose tissue stores), they circulate round the body. Eventually they have to enter the cells and to achieve this you need a particular amino acid called carnitine. You can get this in the diet from animal sources. You can also make it, in your liver, from two other amino acids, methionine and lysine, provided you have eaten these in your diet (they are not ones you can make yourself). This process is helped by iron and vitamin C. If carnitine is in short supply, then the fat keeps circulating, energy is not produced and you will feel unwell, be hungry, but fatigued and have trouble losing weight.

Your liver not only deals with the fats you have eaten, it also converts unwanted proteins and carbohydrates into lipids. This means that when you have eaten too much, be it in the form of fats, proteins or carbohydrates, your liver converts them all into fat that is suitable for storage. This fat is then transported to your adipose (fat) tissues where it forms all those layers of fat you don't want.

By now you will have a growing idea of just how important a healthy liver is, not only to the digestion and metabolism of fats them-selves, but, as a result, to many different aspects of your body and your health, from heart problems to weight loss and energy production.

Proteins

Protein Metabolism

You'll be glad to know that protein metabolism, at the level we will be dealing with it, is a lot less complicated than fat metabolism.

The proteins from your diet are broken down in the intestines into individual amino acids which are then absorbed and transported to the liver. Several things can then happen to them. They can be rebuilt into protein, in the appropriate sequence and structure to make your own human protein, such as muscle protein, liver or heart protein, hair protein etc. They can be changed into different amino acids if these latter ones are needed in greater quantities than were available from food (this is true of some, but not all, amino acids). They can be used to make hormones and other messenger molecules, such as those called 'neurotransmitters' that carry messages from nerve cell to nerve cell or between nerve cell and muscle cell, or they can be broken down, used for energy and disposed of.

The amino acids that are components of the protein you eat fall into two groups. The first group consists of arginine, histidine, iso-leucine, leucine, lysine, methionine, phenylalanine, threonine, tryptophan, valine. It is important that you get these from your diet, as you cannot make them. You may sometimes be prescribed them by your naturopath for this reason. The second group consists of alanine, asparagine, aspartic acid, cysteine, glutamic acid, glycine, proline, serine, tyrosine. Provided your total intake of amino acids is adequate, if any of these in the second group are in short supply, they can be made from spare amounts of any of the others you have eaten. There are certain other amino acids that can be made within the body. They include carnitine, cystine (two molecules of cysteine joined together), glutamine, hydroxylysine, hydroxyproline and taurine and we'll be talking about some of these later.

The reason I list all their names is so we can consider those with particular reference to your liver. The sulphur amino acids, methionine, cysteine and cystine, are very important for your liver *(see below)*. They contain the sulphur needed for the production of taurine, which is one of the amino acids needed to make bile; you will recall that taurocholic acid is one of the bile acids. Methionine is also needed for the synthesis of lecithin, the emulsifying agent that is an important part of bile.

Some, such as phenylalanine and tyrosine, are converted into hormones. Histidine is converted into histamine, the substance produced when you have an allergic reaction. Tryptophan is converted into serotonin, a messenger molecule between nerve cells in the brain, and into melatonin, which is helpful in the treatment of insomnia and depression.

Protein Synthesis

Proteins are made by joining the basic 20 different amino acids together in particular sequences and structures. This occurs in nearly all the cells of your body, but the liver has several particular roles to play.

Nearly 95 per cent of all the proteins found in the blood are synthesised in the liver, the main one being albumin. When your liver becomes unhealthy, albumin synthesis is reduced proportionately and this means that the level of albumin in the blood can be used as a guide to the degree that the liver is damaged or diseased.

The various blood proteins made by the liver are involved in many different roles. They help to maintain a proper fluid balance within the body and prevent fluid retention or oedema. If your liver is faulty and insufficient albumin is made, fluid may leave the blood and enter the tissues, causing the classical swelling, weight gain and other signs of fluid retention. The proteins contribute to the viscosity of the blood (its degree of 'stickiness') and thus to normal blood flow and normal blood pressure, so a lack of these proteins can adversely affect your blood pressure. Also, two of the blood proteins, prothrombin and fibrinogen, are essential for blood clotting.

The liver also makes a variety of carrier proteins that operate within the blood. These are proteins that bind with a variety of substances, helping to carry them through the bloodstream. The substances include fats, vitamins, minerals, hormones and more. Without these proteins, the transport of many substances throughout the body would be compromised.

Amino Acid Breakdown

Eventually all amino acids, just like the fatty acids, are broken down into their individual components, releasing energy in the process, and these are excreted from the body. For all three food groups this means carbon dioxide and water, but unlike fats and carbohydrates, amino acids also contain the amino group and this too has to be eliminated. The way the liver deals with this amino group is critical to your health because even small amounts of ammonia in the blood are highly toxic.

Ammonia reaches the liver in several different ways. Some of it comes from the intestines, where dietary protein is first broken down into amino acids, and then some of these amino acids are broken down further, by gut bacteria, releasing the ammonia. This ammonia travels to the liver via the portal vein and the liver extracts the ammonia. If this is done correctly, when the blood leaves the liver it has virtually no ammonia left in it.

Ammonia is also released from the amino acids in the kidneys. Some of this is excreted directly in the urine, where it is used to balance the amount of acid being excreted. However some of the ammonia produced in the kidneys goes back into the blood and eventually reaches the liver, where it has to be dealt with.

Ammonia is also released by all tissues, following the breakdown of some of the amino acids in them, and carried by the blood to the liver, where it is rapidly taken up so that the blood level of ammonia does not rise above the safety threshold.

All this ammonia is converted, by a healthy liver, into urea, a compound that is very much safer than ammonia. Ammonia in the bloodstream flowing through the brain is highly toxic, urea is not. High levels of ammonia in the urine could damage the kidneys and bladder, urea does not. High levels of ammonia in all tissues can do some damage, urea is much safer for all of them. Your liver clearly has a vital role to play.

If your liver fails and the ammonia level in the blood and brain rises, a range of very unpleasant symptoms can result, mostly stemming from the damage to the brain and nervous system. These include slurred speech, blurred vision, characteristic tremors, brain damage, coma (often called 'hepatic coma' to indicate its cause), and eventually death.

We do not live in a black-and-white world – there are many shades of grey. Thus even if your liver is only slightly sluggish, even if there is only a small increase in the level of circulating ammonia, it is important to keep in mind that ammonia is a toxic substance, and adverse symptoms can result.

Carbohydrates

Types of Carbohyrate

Carbohydrates are a straightforward group of compounds, with a common structure. They are based dominantly on one compound, glucose, and to a lesser extent on two others, fructose and galactose, although there are also a few others, minor in absolute amount in food, though vitally important in your body, that we will not consider here. Two others, ribose and deoxyribose, occur in the nucleic acids of genes RNA and DNA.

As the name implies, carbohydrates are compounds that contain, approximately, an equal number of carbon atoms and water molecules. More usefully they can be thought of as being either simple sugars or else large molecules made up of simple sugars joined together in chains. The simple sugars (monosaccharides) are galactose, glucose and fructose. The double sugars (disaccharides) include table sugar (sucrose, made of glucose and fructose), milk sugar (lactose, made of glucose and galactose) and maltose (made from glucose plus glucose). Starches are much larger and are made by adding hundreds, even thousands of glucose units together; they are found in vegetables, legumes and grains. When the glucose units are put together in a slightly different way they form glycogen, also called animal starch, which is found in the liver and muscles. Then there is fibre, more accurately called 'non-digestible carbohydrate' in this case cellulose. In general it is also made up of thousands of glucose units, but they are put together in such a way that you cannot break them down, only certain gut bacteria can do that, mainly the ones found in the digestive system of cows and other ruminants. Thus fibre survives the digestive tract all the way to the colon, where it can hold water and swell up, thus adding to the bulk of the stool as well as providing necessary food for the colon bacteria (some fibre contains compounds other than glucose, but that is beyond the scope of our discussion here).

Carbohydrate Digestion

With the exception of fibre, carbohydrates are broken down in the digestive tract into glucose. This is absorbed and carried to the liver. Fructose (from table sugar and from fruit) and galactose (from milk) are also carried to the liver and give it another job to do.

Carbohydrate Absorption, Transport and Storage

Glucose travels through the bloodstream with relative ease and its concentration is kept within a narrow range by two groups of hormones: those, such as insulin, that push it into the cells when your blood level rises above normal; and others, such as adrenaline, that bring it out of the cells if your blood level falls below normal. If this mechanism fails and the level falls significantly below normal, or if it remains low for a prolonged period, you become hypoglycaemic, and if it rises and remains high, you become diabetic. The liver has several important roles to play in this process, all of which we will discuss later.

Any glucose that is not needed for immediate energy is converted into fat and stored in your adipose tissues.

Carbohydrate Metabolism

Blood Glucose

Carbohydrates from your diet supply glucose, the blood sugar necessary for your survival. You can get ample amounts of this glucose from starchy foods, vegetables and fruit, so, sad though you may feel it to be, you have absolutely no nutritional need for sugar and sweet things whatsoever. In fact they can do you harm. Not only, unlike the grains and vegetables, do they fail to provide any other nutrients, but they are also absorbed rapidly, hitting your bloodstream in a rush, and this puts severe stress on your mechanisms for keeping your blood sugar level within the acceptable normal range.

Energy Production

Your blood glucose circulates past all the cells in your body and they can call on it as needed for a quick source of energy. When you run a 100-yard dash, jump up suddenly to answer the door bell, or even move a finger, it is your blood glucose that is the energy source. When you do prolonged physical activity, however, it is the stored fats that are mobilised to produce more energy.

Glycogen Storage

While the role the liver plays in carbohydrate metabolism is not quite so critical as the roles it plays in protein and fat metabolism (which, if they fail, can be life-threatening), it is none the less important. Anyone suffering from hypoglycaemia or low blood sugar problems will tell you that the symptoms can be devastating.

A high blood sugar level can also be harmful. When the level does rise above the normal range the liver takes up some of this excess sugar, absorbing it into its own cells and helping to reduce the blood level to within the normal range. This glucose is then converted into glycogen, the 'animal starch' already mentioned. Then when the blood sugar level falls below the normal range the liver mobilises some of this glycogen, breaks it down into individual glucose molecules and releases them into the bloodstream to bring the concentration up to normal.

Benefits of Liver Glycogen

Thus the liver acts as both a storehouse of carbohydrates and a stabiliser of your blood sugar level. This is beneficial for your blood sugar level and energy output, but there are also other, beneficial, consequences. About 5 per cent of the glucose that enters the liver cells is converted into glycogen and if the blood sugar level stays high, the liver glycogen level will remain high. This in turn reduces your liver's ability to remove the amino group from amino acids and so amino acid breakdown is reduced. Thus a diet high in complex carbohydrates can make the protein you eat last longer, a process known as the 'protein-sparing' effect. The high level of glycogen in the liver also prevents the formation of ketones. These are undesirable substances that are made from fats and occur in the urine of diabetics or people who eat an exceptionally low carbohydrate diet. A high level of liver glycogen also helps your liver to deal with toxins.

There is another job for your liver to do. We have talked of blood sugar and glucose as if they are the same thing and in fact they generally are, but there are exceptions. Starchy foods, including grains, legumes and vegetables, break down into thousands of glucose molecules. However when you drink milk the lactose (milk sugar) in it also contains and releases galactose, and when you eat table sugar (sucrose), the kind you buy in the shops and find in sweets and desserts, it also contains and releases fructose. In addition you also get fructose from honey and from many different kinds of fruit. Thus as well as glucose you are absorbing galactose and fructose. These latter two are absorbed and taken to the liver, but there they have to be changed into glucose because, ultimately, this is the type of sugar that all the cells want. If for some reason your liver falls down on the job you can have these two sugars circulating in the bloodstream and causing harm. An excess of fructose, for instance, can be converted into sorbitol and and this can cause problems with the eyes, reducing your vision.

The cells convert glucose into energy via a group of reactions called the Krebs cycle. This is the major source of energy for everything you do. It requires several trace minerals including magnesium and manganese and B group vitamins including B1, B2, B3, B5, lipoic acid and biotin as coenzymes and if they are absent energy production is compromised. A healthy and well nourished liver can store and provide these needed B vitamins. Otherwise, lactic acid will be formed and this can cause problems.

Lactic Acid

The problem with lactic acid is that it cannot be broken down in most cells, only in those of the liver. If, when it arrives, your liver immediately absorbs it and deals with it you will have few problems. However if your liver does not do this, if it is allowed to continue in circulation and build up, it can generate a number of symptoms. These include anxiety, panic, hypertension and chest pains, in fact all the symptoms that could be attributed to an anxiety attack and/or a heart attack.

This can be prevented by supplying the missing coenzymes, vitamin B1, lipoic acid and magnesium. It can be treated in the short term, or palliated, by supplying calcium to combine with the lactic acid. However you should also recognise that the liver has failed in its job of dealing with the lactic acid and so should work on improving the function of your liver.

Vitamins and Minerals

Vitamins A

In addition to the fats, proteins and carbohydrates, many of the trace nutrients also depend on a healthy liver.

Vitamin A is a fat-soluble vitamin and is stored in a healthy liver. When it is needed by other tissues it is shipped out of the liver and sent to its target. Because it is fat soluble, its transport through the blood is not simple. It requires a protein carrier molecule called retinol-binding protein and this is made in the liver with the help of zinc. It is possible that some of the adverse effects of an excessive intake of vitamin A are due to problems with mobilising it from the liver. Thus again, by improving the health and function of your liver you could avoid a potential problem.

B Vitamins

B group vitamins are also stored in the liver. This is, doubtless, largely because the liver needs considerable quantities of them for the many different functions it performs, but it does also mean that in emergencies some of them can be donated to other tissues. Liver storage is particularly important for vitamin B12, by far the largest vitamin and one that is difficult to absorb. A healthy liver can store a sufficient quantity of this vitamin to last for several weeks. Again, your liver needs a readily available supply of this vitamin for the many different jobs it has to do. So it is essential that you provide your liver with a steady supply of all these vitamins, both from your diet and, in all probability, from supplements as well.

Iron and Copper Metabolism

Iron is vital for healthy blood, being part of the red pigment, haemoglobin, that, as most people know, carries oxygen to the tissues. However it plays other roles as well. It is a vital part of the cells' ability to convert food into energy. It is also part of the liver's arsenal of weapons in the fight against toxins, for the synthesis of carnitine and many other reactions. The absorption and transport of iron and copper is dependent on a variety of carrier molecules which, in turn, are dependent on a healthy liver; and a healthy liver can also store significant amounts of these minerals, either for use by the liver itself or elsewhere.

Immune Function

The liver plays a variety of roles in relation to your immune system. By eliminating toxins it reduces some of the work the immune system has to do. By reducing the occurrence of allergic responses, it also gives the immune system less to do. In fact in this regard when you improve the health of your liver you may find a variety of reactions disappearing that either you or your practitioner had attributed either to allergies or to a faulty immune system.

There are special cells within your liver, called Kupffer cells, that play a vital role within the immune system. It is their job to deal with the toxins and unwanted organisms that reach the liver, and to clean up the blood. To do this they move throughout the liver, waving their long slender protrusion into all the nooks and crannies searching for their targets. They absorb the toxins that come in from pollution and the air you breathe, from your food and water supply, from the substances you apply to your body and from any other possible source; they also absorb the toxins made within your body. They deal with these in whatever way is most appropriate, often breaking them down to smaller, safer components which can then be eliminated. In addition they deal with partially digested proteins, potential allergens, unwanted hormones, cancer cells, dead cells and the general detritus that arrives.

These Kupffer cells also absorb the viruses, bacteria, yeasts, moulds, parasites and more that can invade your system and cause harm. They produce a variety of substances that attack these and destroy or kill them and then start to break them down.

However the Kupffer cells can do just so much. If they are overworked, if they are overwhelmed with toxins and pathogens, they just can't cope. Then some of the toxins remain stored in your liver, damaging it and reducing its ability to do all its other jobs, and your blood system becomes, or remains, toxic.

This means that if your liver is unhealthy and your Kupffer cells are overworked you are increasingly likely to get infections, to find that a cold is not clearing up as fast as it does in other people, or that you get repeated bouts of flu without seeming ever to shake them off properly. This is in addition to all the other symptoms that can result from the circulating toxins.

Also, if certain hormones are allowed to remain too long in the blood (a possible result of poor liver function), the amount of white blood cells and antibodies in the blood will fall and so your immune system will be further weakened.

Hormones

As already explained, hormones are substances made in one part of the body and transported to other parts or tissues, where they cause something to happen. The organs that produce hormones are called glands.

So, for example, the adrenal glands produce the adrenal hormones. When you are stressed your adrenal glands are stimulated and they then produce and secrete several of the adrenal hormones which travel through the bloodstream stimulating tissues to cope with the crisis. When you are cold or lacking in energy your thyroid gland is stimulated to produce thyroid hormones that travel through the bloodstream and stimulate the target cells to increase their rate of energy production.

Where do these stimulations come from? Usually from the master glands within the brain: the hypothalamus and the pituitary. They in turn are stimulated by a variety of factors including the nerve input into the brain (such as sights, sounds, touch), your thoughts (anxieties, concerns, and a variety of emotions) and a variety of chemical messengers bringing information back from the body itself (such as temperature, energy production, etc.).

There are two types of hormones, those made from amino acids and those based on the steroid nucleus and derived from cholesterol. As well as being actively involved in amino acid metabolism and in cholesterol metabolism, the liver is also involved with your endocrine or hormonal system.

An important function of the liver in relation to hormones, particularly the steroid ones, is getting rid of them once they have done their job. If this is not done then you will have an excess of these hormones circulating in the bloodstream. So it is valuable to know what these hormones can do and what might happen if they keep circulating.

Protein-Based Hormones

To recap, the amino acids, derived from the proteins in your diet, are carried to the liver via the portal vein. The liver then uses some of them to make proteins and ships others out as amino acids.

One amino acid, tyrosine, makes the hormone thyroxine. This comes in two forms known as T3 and T4. The numbers relate to the number of iodine atoms in the molecule. It is made in the thyroid gland. This gland lies at the centre front of your neck and influences your metabolic rate, dictating how fast and effectively you convert food into energy and heat rather than into body fat. When the gland is underactive you will have insufficient energy, feel the cold and gain weight rapidly. When it is overactive you will be sweating and hungry yet losing weight, but worst of all, you will be uptight, jittery, unable to relax, full of 'go-go' energy that you cannot easily control. Tyrosine can come from your diet. However it can also, if necessary, be made, in the liver, from another amino acid phenylalanine.

Different types of hormones come from the two adrenal glands which sit on top of each of your kidneys. They are made up of two parts, an inner medulla and an outer cortex. They each make hormones, but different types of hormones. The hormones from the medulla are adrenaline and noradrenaline and they, like thyroxine, are made from tyrosine, or, if your liver is willing, from phenylalanine that has been converted into tyrosine.

When you are faced with a sudden stress adrenaline and noradrenaline are released from these glands and go to a variety of tissues, stimulating them into action and triggering the production of sufficient energy to deal with the crisis. Some of it goes back to the liver and instructs that to release some of the stored glycogen and let glucose enter the bloodstream. This glucose flows round your system and provides the other cells with an immediate energy source. It also helps you to maintain a normal blood sugar level and so to avoid the symptoms of hypoglycaemia. If there is insufficient glycogen stored in the liver, or if the liver does not release it, then your ability to respond to stress is reduced. These hormones also stimulate the release of fatty acids from adipose tissues and these too are available for the rapid production of energy. As with all hormones, once the crisis is over you have to get rid of these two hormones or you would be tense and in a permanent state of crisis.

Thyroxine, adrenaline and noradrenaline are small hormones. Other hormones are much larger, for instance parathyroid hormone, which is essential for the proper absorption of calcium from the digestive tract and for keeping blood calcium levels up to normal. Calcitonin has an opposite effect to parathyroid hormone in that it helps to lower your blood calcium level when it is too high and to put that calcium into the bones. Insulin helps to balance your blood sugar level. Glucagon, encourages the mobilisation of glucose from the pancreas in response to a low level of blood sugar.

It is unlikely that your diet provides exactly the right amount of all the amino acids involved and so a considerable amount of juggling may be necessary to ensure you have the correct amount of each one, something of which a healthy liver is eminently capable.

Once these amino acid and protein hormones have circulated throughout your system and done their job they have to be deactivated, and this is another role a healthy liver plays.

Steroid Hormones

The steroid hormones are produced in a number of different tissues and perform a wide range of functions. Like cholesterol, they cannot be broken down in your cells, they have to be eliminated largely intact in the bile, and this can only be done by the liver. If the liver fails to do this correctly then there will be a variety of adverse consequences. So first of all, let's find out what these hormones are and what they do.

The first group comes from the adrenal cortex and so they are often called corticoids. The mineral croticoids, such as aldosterone, act on the transport of mineral electrolytes, elements such as sodium and potassium, and help to control the way water is distributed throughout the body. Aldosterone had a very important job to do in primitive times, before settled farming and processed foods entered our lives, and it is worth taking a moment to think about this. Wild food, that is to say wild animals and fresh fruit, vegetables and seeds, is relatively low in sodium and high in potassium. To maintain a correct balance it was thus evolutionarily important that the body had a way of holding on to the sodium it had and letting potassium be lost in the urine; this is what aldosterone does. An indication of the importance of sodium in the diet is the value of salt throughout the ages; even being at one time a system of currency (hence salary, the amount of salt you had earned).

Now, however, salt is available too freely. The average diet contains much more sodium than potassium and the action of aldosterone, in still clinging on to the sodium in the body, can cause fluid retention, and is likely to create high blood pressure in susceptible people. If your overburdened liver fails to remove any excess of aldosterone then high blood pressure is more likely.

The next layer of the cortex produces the glucocorticoids which affect the metabolism of proteins, fats and carbohydrates and thus affect every cell in your body. They include cortisol (hydrocortisone) and corticosterone. These steroids stimulate the breakdown of proteins and the release of amino acids into the cells in all tissues except the liver, where these amino acids are taken up and converted into glycogen, the storage form of carbohydrate already mentioned. If this process were to continue beyond the appropriate point, it would lead to significant breakdown of body protein and damage to the tissues. If this is happening when you are trying to lose weight, for instance, you will lose muscle tissue, and that is not good, as we shall see later, particularly if you are a yo-yo dieter. It would also lead to periods of abnormally high blood glucose, as found in diabetes. These glucocorticoids also stimulate fat breakdown from the arms and legs and increase its deposition in the face, neck and trunk – the last thing you want if you are trying to look slimmer.

Another serious consequence of raised glucocorticoid levels is that the number of certain types of white blood cell goes down and so does the quantity of antibodies, these are essential components of your immune system so you are more prone to infections and allergies,

The inner layer of the cortex produces the sex hormones in both sexes. These include androgens or male sex hormones such as testosterone and the female sex hormones such as oestrogen. Both sexes need some of the androgens and both need some oestrogens.

In women the ovaries produce two female hormones, oestrogen, and progesterone. These hormones come from different parts of your ovaries and their production peaks at different times of the month, hence the monthly cycle. If this sequence and these levels are upset, such as by the lack of breakdown, a variety of problems, physical and emotional, can arise.

In men, the testes secrete testosterone, and an excess of them can cause problems such as increased body hair and other male characteristics. These steroid hormones are not readily broken down in the body. It is up to the liver to remove them from circulation and then excrete them from the body, somewhat modified, in the bile.

Your Liver as Your Detoxifying Organ

Anywhere in the world, in the twentieth century, human beings are being subjected to a vast increase in toxins, in 'unnatural' chemical and physical challenges to their body and how it functions, compared to that experienced by people in previous centuries. In the industrialised world, and especially in urban settings, the increase is enormous. In fact it is almost certain that we are as yet unaware of much of the damage we are doing. We regularly hear that some drug, food substance, farming practice or industrial waste that was claimed to be safe is, in fact harmful. Sometimes the offending agent or activity is banned, sometimes we are told we just have to live with it. More particularly, your liver has to live with it and to deal with it.

Such toxins include all the chemicals in the food chain, from chemical fertilisers, fungicides, herbicides and pesticides, through the various growth factors, hormones, antibiotics and other drugs used in agriculture to the thousands of chemicals added to foods during processing. These latter include flavours and flavour enhancers, colours, preservatives, solvents, emulsifiers, homogenisers and others, plus further pesticides (such as on dried fruit), glazing agents and setting agents. There are also the myriad chemicals in the water supply, coming from agricultural run-off, industrial sources and all the other factors that drain into the water system; plus the chemicals added to the water in an effort to purify it and the chemicals produced in it as the various components interact. Add to that the environmental and industrial toxins in the atmosphere and the dust that surround us, the fumes from traffic, the chemicals in the home, office and factory, in buildings, furniture, carpets and fabrics, the chemicals produced within air-conditioning units, office chemicals and more. Homes can be particularly toxic places, as you use cleaning sprays, polishes, fabric softeners, ironing sprays, detergents, deodorisers, insect killers and repellents. Then add the various pastes, potions and sprays applied to your own body such as cosmetics, hair sprays and colours, perfumes and deodorants, and substances in and sprayed onto clothing.

In addition to these chemical toxins there are all the physical forces that impact on your body. These include the effects of chemical radiation (radioactivity), electromagnetic fields and others. Examples include neon and fluorescent lights, radio and television waves plus the direct effects that result from sitting in front of a TV, the effects of power lines and pylons, mobile phones and more, much more.

It has been estimated that you take into your body several thousand different chemical substances that are not part of your dietary or nutritional requirements, that are not normally present in the human body, and for which the body has no safe excretory route. You almost certainly have significant quantities of toxins stored throughout your body in such places as the bones and adipose tissues, as well as in the liver itself.

To a large extent it is up to your liver to deal with these toxins. To do this it has several powerful enzyme systems. If you support these, by providing the necessary nutrients, you can assist your liver greatly in its action as a detoxifying organ.

There are two major steps in this detoxification programme – activation and conjugation – and it is important that they happen together, otherwise you can create further problems.

Put simply:

- Activation is the process of getting the toxins out of their storage locations so they can be dealt with and then eliminated. However, because these substances *are* toxins you do not want them to be roaming freely around your body, perhaps entering other tissues, such as the brain, where they can do harm.

- Conjugation is the process that reduces the risk of this happening. Here the toxins are 'conjugated' or combined with other substances such that the total complex is less dangerous than the toxin itself and can be eliminated from the body causing minimal damage.

Before the dangerous nature of the current toxins was fully recognised, and the need for these two processes to occur in tandem became clear, the traditional naturopathic method of detoxification was fasting, or spending a few days just drinking fruit and vegetable juices. This worked well in the past, when the toxins around were less lethal, when the person had perhaps overindulged in food and drink and led a sedentary life but was not overburdened with a load of chemical drugs and toxins, and affected by physical forces on the body such as electromagnetic fields, radiation and so forth. With time, however, this fasting process came to be accompanied by some unpleasant symptoms such as headaches, nausea, furry tongue, fatigue and a general feeling of being unwell. This was commonly called a 'healing crisis' or a 'detox reaction' and was welcomed as a sign that you did indeed have toxins to eliminate and that you were getting the desired result.

Now, with a greater understanding of the metabolic biochemistry of the body, we can recognise that the toxins had indeed been mobilised or activated, but not conjugated, and we also now know what can be done to induce this conjugation and make the process safer.

To use another analogy, think about the dangers we now face with asbestos, used for a while in the roofs of houses. We now know it is dangerous. To remove it, however, we don't simply rip it out, piling it up on the stairs and sweeping it down to the backdoor and into the dustbin, letting the dust fly everywhere (activation). We recognise its dangers and do it carefully so that the dust and particles are contained, are wrapped in containers and carried out in such a way that the rest of the house does not become impregnated (conjugation and elimination).

This is what has to be done within your body as well, and you rely on a healthy and active liver to accomplish this job. Fortunately it does have some support, as these reactions can also occur, to a certain extent, in the walls of your intestines. However your liver bears the brunt of the work so make sure you give it all the foods and nutrients it needs to accomplish *both* steps.

One of the problems of the fasting method of detoxifying was that the regime did not include protein because it was thought that this gave the digestive system and the liver extra work to do. We now know that protein is essential, daily, and that if you do not have it then the demands of your body are at least partially met by using the protein your liver contains, to the detriment of this organ, and this is obviously not helpful. This is why you will find that the Liver Detox Plan contains protein foods from the start, in the form of fish, initially extending as you progress to other protein sources.

Activation

There is an important enzyme in the liver, cytochrome p450, that plays a vital role in dealing with toxins by oxidising them into forms that are water soluble and that can be transported out of the body. The enzymes involved in this activation need a variety of coenzymes to function at their best. These include vitamins B2, B3 and B6 and the minerals iron, magnesium, manganese, molybdenum and zinc.

Unwanted bi-products of these reactions include highly reactive oxygen free radicals that could, if not dealt with, cause the production of other very reactive and possibly even more toxic substances. To avoid the build-up of free radicals and to reduce this risk of unwanted oxidation side-effect you need additional amounts of the antioxidant nutrients, vitamins A, C and E, beta-carotene, flavonoids, proanthocyanidins and selenium. Beta-carotene has both anti-viral and anti-tumour properties. Silymarin, or milk thistle, is an excellent antioxidant herb to use at this time as it also has a particularly protective effect on the liver. You can also use dandelion as a supporting herb.

Conjugation

The next step is to join these activated substances to small polar molecules and so render them safer. These molecules include cysteine, glucuronic acid, glutathione, glycine, methionine and sulphate. Some of these your body can make for itself, while others must be supplied by your diet. For these conjugating molecules to do their job properly you need vitamins B6, B9 (folic acid) and B12, and the minerals magnesium and selenium. If any of these substances are not available, then further free-radical damage can occur, particularly in the liver. Fortunately they are all commonly available as or in supplements.

If you have only limited amounts of the nutrients needed for both steps, the detoxification process will be slow. Your health will begin to improve, but you will still experience some of the symptoms, though possibly with less severity, while it is going on. If you have the nutrients necessary for step one but not for step two, problems can occur. But if you provide all the nutrients your body needs for both activation and conjugation to go ahead rapidly, you will achieve a rapid detoxification with minimal side-effects. In a few days you will feel a noticeable difference, you will *feel* less toxic. Some patients do describe it as feeling 'clean', as if their system has had a real clear-out.

Clearly the obvious and most sensible route to follow is to change your diet and lifestyle, thus reducing the toxins you are taking in, *and* to take the appropriate supplements so that you can eliminate the toxins already spread throughout your body. Improving your diet, on its own, is unlikely to give you the additional amounts of nutrients you need to deal with past sins.

Your liver has additional ways of dealing with toxins. We have already seen, for instance, that a variety of compounds are produced in the body when there is a job of work for them to do, and that once that job is done, then they must be disposed of. Hormones are a good example. The adrenaline and noradrenaline produced when you are in a stressful situation or an emergency arises, must be got rid of once that situation has passed. This job is done in the liver, which causes them to combine with vitamin C to make adrenascorbate and noradrenascorbate respectively. In the absence of sufficient vitamin C, or if the liver is not performing properly then two other compounds are formed instead, called adrenachrome and noradrenachrome. These are toxic and can cause psychiatric problems, including the symptoms of schizophrenia. Thus vitamin C becomes an important nutrient to enable the liver to deal with waste or 'spent' compounds.

Your Liver's Capacity to Heal Itself

During its lifetime, your liver takes on a lot of challenges. It deals with compounds that can harm it, it gives up some of its protein when there is a need for it, it stores substances, even if they are toxic, when it can do nothing else with them. It is beaten up by the alcohol you drink, challenged by the effect of sugar on your blood sugar level and risks being overburdened when you eat a high-fat diet. Yet your liver is a very forgiving organ. To a limited extent, and provided you give it all the nutrients it needs for repair and rejuvenation, it will do all it can to rebuild itself.

This thought is offered as a word of encouragement, in case you are feeling overwhelmed by what the liver has to do, or in case you feel you have already done so much harm there is little hope. There *is* hope. Your liver wants nothing so much as to help you get better and if you stick to the Liver Detox Plan you can help it to achieve this goal for you.

Part IV

What Harms your Liver

Alcohol

Alcohol, as we know it in a social context, is just one of many hundreds of different alcohols that either exist naturally or can be synthesised. The alcohol that you drink is called ethanol. Meths, another familiar alcohol, is properly called methanol. In fact the ending -ol usually indicates that the substance is an alcohol.

Nearly all alcohols are harmful. Methanol, for instance, may provide the alcoholic with a cheap drink but it will damage the liver even faster than ethanol. However for the rest of this section we will use the word 'alcohol' to mean ethanol.

Alcohol is a carbohydrate, supplying considerable amounts of energy (calories) when it is broken down. 10 mls of ethanol, for instance, supplies approximately 70 calories. This means that if you drink wine that is 12.5 per cent alcohol, 100 ml will give you nearly 90 calories.

When you drink alcohol it is absorbed rapidly and transported to the liver, which has the major job of reducing its toxicity, breaking it down and dealing with the consequences. To do this your liver needs zinc to work with an enzyme called alcohol dehydrogenase. Your liver first converts the alcohol into a compound called acetaldehyde, which unfortunately often causes more symptoms than the alcohol itself, and then further breaks it down until it is fully converted into carbon dioxide and water – what a fate for something that gave you so much pleasure.

Alcohol damages the liver and so does the acetaldehyde. If your liver is faulty and the alcohol and acetaldehyde accumulate, you can both prolong the feeling of being drunk and the symptoms of a hangover, while also, of course, increasing the damage these compounds do to your liver.

Alcohol also increases the amount of fat in your liver. It does this by increasing the amount of fatty-acid-binding-protein, or FABP, and this is what leads to the fatty liver of the heavy drinker. A high level of fat in the liver will both give the liver itself a lot more work to do and leave it less able to fulfil its other obligations.

It has been suggested that your liver can process the equivalent of two glasses of wine a day. In that case two glasses of wine is all you should drink in any one day. Do not tell yourself that since you have had nothing to drink all week you can have 14 glasses at the weekend and all will be well. Think what would happen if the tidal flow stopped for five days and then you suddenly had a high tide that was five times the normal height. There would be an enormous amount of flooding and damage all along the coast. Keep the alcohol tide in your liver down and you can continue to enjoy one or two drinks (and no more) without doing too much harm. Otherwise, alcohol will definitely damage your liver, and seriously. Even if you keep your intake down to this level you would be wise to recognise that it does make extra demands on your liver and to take appropriate action to support it, as described in the Liver Detox Plan.

While on the subject of alcoholic drinks, it is worth considering the merits of the different types. It seems clear that wine is less harmful than the other types and there are several possible reasons for this.

The case for wine

- Wine (no more than two glasses) stimulates the flow of digestive juices thus improving your digestion of an accompanying meal. More than two glasses, as we have seen, would overburden the liver and it would also dilute the digestive juices. It is wise not to drink a large quantity of liquid with a meal for this reason.
- Wine, particularly red wine, contains compounds called proanthocyanidins or OPCs. These are part of the bioflavonoid group which is sometimes referred to as part of a vitamin C complex since they work with vitamin C and often occur in similar foods. They are strong, protective antioxidants which help to protect your heart, brain, eyes, joints and many other tissues and boost the function of your immune system. Two particularly rich sources of these compounds are pine bark and grape seeds.
- White wine is made by extracting the juice from the grapes (red or white) and immediately separating it from the solids that are left behind; thus it contains relatively little of the OPCs. Red wine, on the other hand, is made by crushing the grapes and leaving the juice in contact with the seeds (crushed) and skin. During this time the liquid not only absorbs the red colour from the skin (partly due to OPCs there), but also absorbs the OPCs from the seeds. (If you are a teetotaller do not be concerned, you can probably get about the same amount of OPCs from red grape juice. This is really just an excuse

for the drinker to enable them to feel there is some benefit from red wine to set off the disadvantages of the alcohol!)

- You can also make a case for drinking a glass of wine with a meal in that is generally slows down the rate at which you consume the meal, and this is beneficial to your digestive system.
- Beer, on the other hand, provides an excess of yeast which can disrupt your intestinal flora if you are prone to candidiasis and it severely dilutes your digestive juices if you drink it near to mealtimes.
- Drinking spirits often means you are drinking quantities of soft drinks as well (tonic, ginger ale, coke, etc.) and they do not deliver any OPCs.
- Finally, for many people, it is socially and emotionally disruptive to give up alcohol altogether. This is not always a valid reason for doing something that can have harmful effects, but alcohol can possibly be excused on this basis. Social life and communication are important and, in our society, alcohol has become a significant part of these for many people. Few couples, for instance, will sit down after a hard day's work and have a worthwhile chat over a glass of orange juice. Better the possible damage of a glass of wine than a divorce resulting from lack of communication.

However, if you do drink, be sure to do it in moderation only and to follow the Liver Detox Plan on an ongoing basis.

Cigarettes

The dangers of smoking are well known and now the dangers of passive smoking are also being recognised. Claims have been made that nicotine is not carcinogenic and this may be true *but* – and it is a big but – in its effort to process and eliminate the nicotine and the tar, your body actually converts them into a series of compounds via reactions called hydroxylations, and it is these hydroxylated products that may be causing much of the damage and that may be carcinogenic. It may seem unwise that your body encourages these reactions, just as it may seem unwise that your liver converts alcohol into the possibly more toxic acetaldehyde, but you have to make allowances for the fact that it has only had a few hundred years to learn how to deal with these toxins, a mere nothing against the perspective of our evolution of hundreds of thousands, or even millions of years. As it is, both the original compounds and those that are created have to be dealt with by the liver, so why not give it a fair go – give up smoking, avoid passive smoke and start on the Liver Detox Plan.

Fats

We all know cream is bad, but isn't it delicious? Yet you will now know that a high-fat intake can give your liver a lot of work to do, so if you are going to eat a high-fat diet, make sure you give it all the nutrients it needs so it can perform to its best for you. Ideally, you should aim to moderate your fat intake. Be particularly careful to avoid the trans fatty acids, the ones produced by hydrogenating vegetable oils to make margarine and when fats are heated to a high temperature.

You will find that the Liver Detox Plan allows you to use olive oil for cooking. It is a good idea to use this on bread as well. The Italians do it and it does indeed spread – all you need to do is to pour it onto the knife and then wipe this across the bread. Alternatively use avocado or tahini. If you insist on butter, use it only sparingly. And before you buy *any* spread, be it margarine or some other type, read the label carefully and don't buy it unless it says it contains no hydrogenated fats.

Sugar

In evolutionary times a sweet tooth provided some benefits:

- Most of the poisonous plants taste bitter, so a sweet tooth tended to keep people away from them.
- Fruit, the sweetest food available, is a rich source of vitamin C, an important nutrient. The collection of many kinds of fruit, however, meant climbing trees. The effort might not have been deemed worth it, compared to collecting vegetables from ground level, without the anticipation of the sweet taste.
- Also, fruit contains a high water content and may not have been the food of choice when you were hungry, without the incentive of the sugar it contains.

Now, however, sugar is available in foods other than fruit and so does not confer these benefits. It is too readily available and can cause problems for a number of reasons:

- It supplies 'empty' calories. In other words, it gives you calories but no nutrients that you need.
- It is rapidly absorbed and so hits the bloodstream in a rush. This puts an enormous strain on your blood sugar balancing mechanism and increases your risk of developing either hypoglycaemia or diabetes.

- The metabolism of this sugar requires many nutrients, including vitamins B1, B2, B3, B5, biotin, lipoic acid, copper, iron, magnesium, manganese and zinc, yet it does not provide them, so it actually *reduces* your level of these nutrients available for other purposes in your body.
- It leads to more work for your liver. You have, for instance, a higher output of hormones for the liver to deal with. When your blood sugar falls, as it does following a high intake, your liver has to pump out glucose from its stored glycogen, then take it up again later as the level rises. It also has to deal with the extra hormone produced.

What can you do? Obviously you should give up sugar, but few people have found will-power alone a sufficient tool to accomplish this. Creating a healthy liver is an important step, so is supplying all the nutrients mentioned above. In addition, many people find that if they take a very strong B complex supplement (50 to 100 mg of each vitamin) and some additional vitamin B1, say another 100 mg, their craving for sugar diminishes. Glutamine also helps to reduce sugar cravings.

Drugs: Social, Recreational and Medicinal

All drugs provide a challenge to the liver. Alcohol and cigarettes have already been mentioned. Coffee, tea and chocolate also present problems. It is not just the caffeine (present in all of them) that the liver has to deal with, but also other compounds such as theophylline (in tea) and theobromine (in tea and chocolate). These three compounds are methyl xanthines and are thought to increase the risk of fibrocystic breast disease, birth defects and pancreatic cancer. Coffee contains a variety of compounds, other than caffeine, that can be toxic, so even drinking decaffeinated coffee is not a good idea.

Other recreational drugs, such as marihuana and the harder drugs, put a huge load on the liver. This is not the place to go into all the various side-effects they can cause. Suffice it to say that if you have been taking them you will surely be in need of and benefit from the Liver Detox Plan. If you are still taking them, but want to have the best possible health, you should stop.

Medical drugs have their place – mainly, as one wag put it, in their bottle. However there are times when health has deteriorated to a point that emergency action with drugs is necessary. Generally the need for such drugs is grossly overestimated by the medical profession and occasionally underestimated by some natural therapists. The vast majority of health problems will respond favourably to improvements in diet and lifestyle, accompanied by appropriate supplementation and, if remedies are necessary, by herbal and homoeopathic remedies.

If you are seriously interested in restoring your health, a consultation with a natural therapist could help you to rationalise what you are doing and reduce your intake of medical drugs. However you should also consult with whoever prescribed those drugs. If your doctor is opposed to natural approaches to healthcare, perhaps you can find one who is willing to help and who will co-operate with your naturopath. Many times the naturopathic approach is to improve your health first, then suggest that you may no longer need the drugs you are on. If, for instance, your can improve your health such that your blood pressure returns to normal, even your doctor is likely to agree that you no longer need to take antihypertensive drugs.

Whatever your strategy, it is important that you realise that there is not a single drug medication that does not, in addition to whatever perceived benefits it offers, cause some unwanted and adverse side-effects (toxic reactions). It also, finally, has to be metabolised by your liver and removed from your body. All medical drugs increase the burden on your liver and need the resources of activation and conjugation described above.

Toxins

As already mentioned, the number of toxins to which you are exposed is huge, but don't panic. There are many ways to help your liver cope with them. First, do all you can to avoid and limit your intake of toxins – learn where they are and discover all the ways you can of avoiding them. Second, do all you can, as described in this programme, to detoxify your body and be kind to your liver.

Free Radicals

One of the things that many of both the chemical toxins and the physical hazards we face every day have in common is the development of free radicals, and a brief word of explanation about them is appropriate.

Our world is made up of atoms, slightly over 100 of them. These are combined into larger groupings called molecules. Molecules can also combine to form the very much larger, complex molecules. These are, in fact, what we have been talking about when we talk of fatty acids, glucose, or an amino acid such as methionine (molecules) and starch, glycogen and proteins (macro molecules).

When such molecules break down they generally either split into smaller molecules or they split into two different ions. Ions have a charge and when two are formed from one molecule one of them has a positive charge and one has a negative charge. The molecules that are produced in this way are stable. The ions are less so and each one tends to go looking for a partner of the opposite charge. These reactions happen relatively quickly, but in a controlled way.

Free radicals are different. They are formed when a molecule is torn into two or more pieces in such a way that the parts are neither smaller molecules nor simple ions. They may be charged or not, but they are highly unstable. They are also non-selective in looking for something onto which they can join and, in the process can break up and destroy or damage thousands of other molecules.

Free radicals are extremely dangerous and destructive compounds and it is important that you do all you can to avoid them and, if you are exposed to them, to guard against them. In general they are formed as a result of oxidising reactions, and for this reason your protection from them is achieved by a generous intake of antioxidant nutrients, the most important of which include vitamins A, C and E, beta-carotene and the bioflavonoids, particularly the OPCs and the minerals selenium, zinc, manganese and copper.

Part V

What Goes Wrong

Your liver has amazing powers of self-preservation, and this is fortunate, as most people treat their livers shamefully. This means, however, that when there are obvious symptoms that indicate your liver has begun to fail, this is just the tip of the iceberg and you have probably been overloading it for a considerable time.

Your Liver and Digestion

Because your liver and its partner, your gall bladder, play such a critical role in digestion, particularly fat digestion, it is hardly surprising to find that when your liver begins to fail you develop a number of symptoms related to indigestion or mal-digestion. They manifest throughout the whole digestive tract, even though the liver's actions only really start down in the small intestine. There are a variety of reasons for this and a variety of unpleasant symptoms.

Bad Breath

Bad breath is unpleasant for you; it is also unpleasant for other people and it is socially embarrassing.

If you suffer from this problem the first obvious step to take is to clean your teeth thoroughly, have any holes fixed and improve your overall oral health. Bacteria or parasites lurking in the mouth, in the gums or between the teeth, can produce a variety of reactions that can lead to unpleasant smells and tastes. You should also improve the health of your gums, something that will happen automatically as you follow the Liver Detox Plan.

Bad breath can also be a sign of more complex problems and so before you can improve the situation you may have to look more closely at its possible causes.

To understand what is happening it is important for you to know that smell is caused by individual molecules of the substance in question. They attach to your 'smell receptors' at the back of your nasal

passages and when you taste a food what is actually happening is that
you are smelling it as it passes these sites. This means that if you can
smell or taste some of the food that has just gone down the tubes, some
of it has physically come back up again in the form of tiny air-borne
molecules. However what comes back up may not actually be what
caused the problem.

Consider the question of the gas itself. Few foods actually cause gas,
yet you may have gas in your stomach. One source of this gas is the air
trapped within the foods you eat. When you think of the way most
people gulp their food, how little attention is paid to chewing, and how
often you are talking, walking or doing some physical activity while you
eat, it is hardly surprising to find that many people swallow a considerable amount of air. Some of this is swallowed as a result of gulping the
food, some of it is trapped within the food itself. In a mouthful of hur-
riedly swallowed salad leaves, or gassy white bread, for instance, there
is bound to be some trapped air. This will only be excluded if you have
chewed your food very thoroughly indeed.

As your food is dealt with by the stomach this air is released
and can travel back up the oesophagus. Most of the time it is odourless
and you are not aware that this is happening (except, of course, in obvious situations such as when you have drunk fizzy drinks and these have
lead to one or more obvious burps). The problem starts when foods that
contain aromatic or strongly flavoured compounds are eaten and some
of these flavours are carried up on the ascending air. Because these
substances *are* aromatic they *do* have a flavour and so when they move
past your smell receptors they are recognised and the food from which
they come is then wrongly blamed for causing the gas itself.

The worst group of compounds in this regard are those that contain
aromatic compounds that include sulphur. This is why the cabbage
family, the onion and garlic family and even sweet peppers are often
blamed for bad breath. The answer is not to stop eating those foods,
particularly as they are all exceptionally nutritious, but to improve the
way you chew and eat your food and to improve your digestion.

Another source of gas results from indigestion in the stomach,
brought about largely by an inadequate amount of stomach acid, and
the resultant lack of proper digestion and the possible overgrowth or
unwanted organisms.

The second aspect of the problem brings us back to your liver
and relates to the processes of digestion beyond the stomach, in the
duodenum and small intestine. If your liver and gall bladder are lazy
and the fats in your diet are not properly homogenised in your duodenum, problems develop for two main reasons. First the fat itself is not

properly broken down and digested, so undigested fat remains and can cause problems. You feel bilious and start to say that fats 'disagree' with you. Second, this fat, by coating the other foods, proteins, carbohydrates, fruit and vegetables etc., reduces the ability of enzymes to get at these food particles and they too are not properly broken down. All this undigested food leads to a variety of harmful bacteria and a number of inappropriate chemical reactions start to occur leading to the production of toxins and other unwanted chemicals and to gases.

From the duodenum it is still a relatively short distance back up through the stomach and oesophagus and into the mouth and it is a much greater distance down the whole length of the small and large intestines. So, some of these compounds may come back up the digestive tract and are expelled on your breath, giving it an unpleasant odour. Obviously, from this point of view, the answer to bad breath is to improve your digestion at this level too, and this may well mean following the Liver Detox Plan.

There is yet another way in which you may develop bad breath and this also involves your liver. If you have consumed a range of toxins and the liver cannot deal with them, some of them may be released back into the digestive tract as the liver tries to get rid of them via the stool. You may also try to eliminate some of them via the lungs and, if they have a taste or smell, when you breathe out you will become aware of them.

Treat your liver properly, follow the Liver Detox Plan and you need never have this embarrassing problem again.

Indigestion

The term 'indigestion' applies to faults in *any* part of the digestive system, although some people use it exclusively to describe heartburn (in the area behind and under the base of your sternum or central chest bone) and pain in the stomach, tucked in under your left rib cage. This means that it includes a number of problems that can occur in the abdomen and in the small and large intestines, as well is in your stomach. In a sense we have already considered this when talking about bad breath. Liver problems and lack of bile can lead to failure of proper fat digestion and reduced stimulus of the pancreas to produce digestive enzymes. The way this interferes with the digestion of both fats and the rest of your food can lead to nausea and vomiting, abdominal bloating and distension, wind and even more severe problems such as spastic colon and irritable bowel syndrome. This may all lead to a loss of appetite, though sadly (for most people) this rarely leads to loss of weight.

Indigestion resulting from poor liver function can also lead to irritation of the intestinal wall and a leaky gut. This in turn can lead to increased absorption of toxins, further enlarging the load on your liver, and the absorption of partially digested food and hence allergies, thus challenging your immune system and, again, your liver. It can also reduce your absorption of essential nutrients, particularly the minerals that need the carrier molecules in a healthy intestinal mucosa to ensure their proper absorption and transport. It can also worsen any problems you may have that are related to candida, as the disturbed conditions in the digestive tract tend to favour their growth and expansion over and above that of the more desirable healthy bacteria. You then have not only their direct effects, but also the increased absorption of the toxins they produce, through the leaky gut.

Another result of these problems may be either diarrhoea or constipation, which brings us to the final part of the digestive tract.

Constipation and Diarrhoea

Constipation

Most people think they are 'regular' if they 'go once a day – or most days, anyway', as patients frequently put it to me, when in fact they mean that they go about four or fives times a week. Yet this is not enough. Think about it. You eat three times a day – more if you have snacks in between meals. This means that there is rubbish to process three (or more) times a day. Yes indeed, I do mean that you should 'go' about three times a day.

So you may have been told, all your life, and even by your doctor, that once a day, usually after breakfast, is sufficient, but this may just mean that your doctor is constipated too. What we do know is that in communities where the diet has a much higher fibre content, such as those in rural Africa or Asia, three or more large, bulky, soft (mushy) stools a day are common. This on its own might not mean much, but when you learn that such societies can have as little as 5 per cent of the incidence of irritable bowel syndrome, colitis, diverticulitis, haemorrhoids and other bowel problems, including bowel cancer, compared to people in this country, I think you will agree that this would seem to be a good idea.

To prevent constipation, fibre is needed to increase the bulk of your stool. This is provided in the Liver Detox Plan in the form of slippery elm powder, psyllium hulls and linseed, as well as by the fact that you are encouraged to eat a lot more in the way of vegetables and fruit, and to replace refined grains, such as white flour and rice, with their wholemeal equivalents. However fibre is not the only requirement – you also need water. You should aim to drink about one and a half litres of water a day. In addition, the greater amounts of fruit and vegetables you will be eating will help lead to a satisfactory fluid intake.

Back to your liver, since it too has an important part to play in normalising your bowel function. This is because bile, produced by the liver and stored in the gall bladder, has a stimulating effect on peristaltic action. Peristalsis is the undulating flow of contractions and relaxations of the muscles along the walls of your digestive system that propels the waste material along the intestinal tract.

Many of the herbs in the detox programme are cholagogues, substances that stimulate the function of the gall bladder, and they have a gentle laxative effect. Note here that the important thing is to stimulate the liver and gall bladder. Do not be tempted to take laxatives such as senna or cascara, or even medical laxatives. These may simply irritate the intestinal lining, cause a flurry of activity and then lead to exhausted tissues and to further constipation and a dependence on laxatives for any movement to occur at all. The answer to constipation is the Liver Detox Plan. By the time you have been on it for a few weeks or months, you will almost certainly find the situation is improving.

Diarrhoea

In my early days in practice I was concerned when patients came back after a short period during which they had followed the suggestions I had given them, saying they now had diarrhoea. Then I discovered that to their minds, anything more than one hard motion a day was diarrhoea. Normal motions, i.e. three large and mushy stools a day, they wrongly labelled diarrhoea. This taught me that education was a vital aspect of naturopathic healing and so it is worth repeating here that three large and soft stools each day is perfectly natural. In fact you should probably go as often as you eat, since you are dealing with something approximating a continuous conveyor belt.

Diarrhoea is not so much a matter of going frequently as of having stools that are unformed or liquid. There can be several reasons for this, but they are beyond the scope of this book. An obvious consequence of diarrhoea, however, is that food passes through the gut so fast that nutrients are not properly absorbed. Ironically, the solution to this problem is often the same as the solution to constipation, namely, eat more fibre, particularly the soluble forms, as instructed in the Liver Detox Plan. Fibre, as we have seen, is simply complex carbohydrates that are not broken down in the small intestine and so survive intact into the colon. By their nature they absorb water and swell up. This normally *keeps* sufficient water in the colon, rather than allowing it to be absorbed back into the body and leaving the stool to dry up. When there is *too much* water in the stool the extra fibre will help to 'set' it, rather like a jelly. The movement then slows down and normalises.

Gall Bladder Problems

If you find yourself saying that you can't digest fatty foods, or that rich foods upset you, the problem may be caused by your gall bladder as well as or instead of your liver.

You will recall that your gall bladder produces the bile that is essential for fat digestion. If there is an obstruction to this flow, no matter how hard your liver works you will still have digestive problems.

Inflammation

An early problem that can occur is inflammation of the mucous membrane lining the gall bladder. This is called cholecystitis. It is the most common gall bladder problem. You may have no symptoms from this, or you may experience localised pain over the gall bladder, or you may experience pain that radiates through to your back in the area of the base of your right shoulder blade. The pain can vary from a mild feeling of unease to an extreme pain. You may feel it intermittently, particularly after a meal rich in fats, or in bed at night, or it may be there much of the time.

Gallstones

Gallstones are another common problem and are often the cause of the inflammation. It is thought that about 10 per cent of the total population, or 20 per cent of people over 40 years of age, have gallstones, often without knowing it.

What are gallstones? They are accretions of solid material that form within the gall bladder. They may be made of different ingredients, may be large or small, there may be many or only one, and they may form for a number of reasons. They can be present and yet lead to no symptoms, so that you remain unaware of them, or they can cause a variety of symptoms varying from mild to severe. If they move down the duct and become stuck they can, particularly when you eat a fatty meal, become excruciatingly painful.

Precipitates and stones may be formed by a combination of calcium and bilirubin caused by a local bacterial infection. Because there is calcium in this type of stones they can be detected by X-rays.

The most common type of gallstone, however, occurring in 85 per cent of cases, is made mainly of cholesterol and cholesterol derivatives. These stones do not contain calcium and they are not detected by X-rays, but they can be picked up by ultrasound. How do they form? As we have seen, bile contains a small amount of free cholesterol. If the amount of cholesterol rises, or the amount of lecithin or bile salts fall, then the cholesterol becomes insoluble and is likely to precipitate and form stones.

Two factors are important here. First, a high-fat diet, as we have seen, stimulates cholesterol synthesis in the small intestines so can lead to an increase of cholesterol. So to prevent this type of gallstone, or to help to improve the situation, the answer is to eat less fat. Second, since lecithin helps to keep this type of stone in solution, lecithin should be added to your diet. On its own, this will not necessarily solve the problem, but it could help.

In any discussion of gallstones it is worth repeating that many, many people have stones without knowing about them. These so-called 'silent stones' may have been there for years without producing any symptoms. They may discovered by accident, during an X-ray or ultrasound investigation for some other problem. They may only be discovered during a post-mortem, having caused no symptoms throughout the person's life.

If you do have them, once they are discovered an enthusiastic surgeon may advise having them removed immediately. A more cautious practitioner may advise doing nothing, provided they cause no adverse symptoms, such as pain or floating stool, pale coloured stools or stools that contain fat, and so long as they don't seem to be interfering with digestion. If you do have stones and if you choose the latter option, then put into practice the ideas given in this book for improving liver and gall bladder function and you may well find that they diminish.

If you do choose to have gallstones removed, perhaps because you have some symptoms you attribute to them, a word of warning is in order. Many people find that, relatively soon after the operation, they develop 'post-cholecystectomy syndrome', a group of symptoms very similar to those they had before the operation. These symptoms may be caused by some stones that were left behind, by new stones that form or by stones caught in the duct. However it is also possible that the stones that were there were actually silent and not causing the symptoms at all, and that the symptoms were related to other problems related to bile flow and function, in which case, removal of the stones could not be expected to improve the situation.

There can be another problem. There have been reports of increased incidence of right-sided colon cancer in people who have had their gall bladder removed. It has been postulated that this is due to the continuous trickle of bile from the liver (since there is no gall bladder to store it) and its accumulation at the beginning of the ascending colon.

Lost your Gall Bladder?

The problem with having your gall bladder removed as the major form of treatment is that you have done nothing to correct the situation that caused the original problem. It's a bit like getting rid of the dustbin because it is found to be full of rubbish each week – you haven't solved the problem of the rubbish itself.

So, after the operation, the work of the gall bladder still has to be done. Bile still has to be made, it still flows down the hepatic duct and it is still needed in the small intestine for the digestion of fat. It is also still possible for stones to form, particularly if this duct has tended to expand and form a pouch. So, if you have already suffered from gallstones and have had your gall bladder removed, it is still important to pay attention to your liver and gall bladder and to follow the Liver Detox Plan. You continue to need bile and you want it to be of the correct composition and you want it to flow correctly, both of which will result if you follow the plan.

Major Liver Diseases

So far we have considered semi-serious liver problems, albeit ones with possibly serious consequences, ranging in severity from so mild that although you may have a few generalised symptoms absolutely nothing shows up when your doctor does the regular blood tests to something that is more obvious with, for instance, raised liver enzymes in a blood test and some fairly severe symptoms. There are, however, some major liver problems that are extremely serious and potentially life-threatening. These too can be helped by the Liver Detox Plan, followed by a programme of nutrients to rebuild the liver and restore its function. However, in such cases, you should also be working with a practitioner who fully understands the seriousness of the problems and can provide authoritative help.

Cirrhosis

In cirrhosis there is significant structural damage to the liver and as a result its function is impaired and a variety of health problems arise.

The most common cause is alcohol consumption and in Americans between 45 and 65 years of age it is the fourth leading cause of death following heart disease, cancer and strokes. As with fatty livers, there may be very few symptoms until the damage is extensive. Eventually such generalised symptoms as fatigue, weakness, reduced libido and a general feeling of unwellness can occur.

So if you drink alcohol and cannot claim to feel absolutely 100 per cent healthy, the Liver Detox Plan could be part of your insurance policy for a healthy liver. If you have cirrhosis you will benefit from the Liver Detox Plan plus a high protein intake, up to about 70 gm – a day, and additional amounts of vitamin B1. You should also, of course, stop drinking alcohol or taking drugs.

Fatty Liver

Fatty liver can be caused by a wide range of drugs and chemical toxins including alcohol and carbon tetrachloride, and drugs such as steroids and antibiotics. It occurs when fats build up in the liver and are dispersed throughout it and the liver becomes larger in size.

Although this is a severe condition and can be fatal it often gives no signs or symptoms until very far advanced. Sometimes there may be local tenderness, difficulty in metabolising fats and easy weight gain.

Treatment for this must obviously focus on any possible cause, such as the toxins listed above. You should avoid alcohol, lose weight (if necessary) and follow the Liver Detox Plan with the additional inclusion of 1,000 mcg of folic acid daily.

Hepatitis

Hepatitis means, literally, 'inflammation of the liver'. There are several types, generally (though not only) caused by viruses, alcohol and drugs. They are all serious, they are all variously infectious and, if you have the disease, you will doubtless already be under medical care. Whatever you are doing, in that regard, should be continued. The Liver Detox Plan can readily be added on to your present treatment, however you would be well advised to discuss it fully with your practitioner.

Jaundice

Jaundice is a yellow coloration of the skin and mucous membranes caused by an excessive amount of bilirubin, which is produced by the liver and, inadvertently, able to circulate through the bloodstream. Let's find out how this occurs.

When the hepatic duct, from the liver to the gall bladder and duodenum, or the cystic duct from the gall bladder directly to the duodenum, become blocked or constricted, bile flow is obstructed. This leads to the bile moving into the bloodstream instead. As the bile pigments build up in the bloodstream this becomes yellowed, as do the tissues through which it flows. Thus you get the yellow coloration of the skin, eyes and mucous membranes which is typical of jaundice.

Other causes of jaundice include an excessive breakdown of haemoglobin, which can lead to both anaemia and to an excess amount of bilirubin. If the liver does not take up the bilirubin, it remains in circulation, and if the liver does not properly convert it into bile pigments, or if, once created, too much of the bile pigment is diverted back into the blood instead of to the gall bladder, jaundice will also result. Notice, however, that all these causes, essentially, refer back to problems with the liver, and the solution to all of them is to improve liver function and stimulate the flow of bile to the gall bladder.

Some people who consume a lot of carotene-rich foods, such as carrot and carrot juice and other strongly coloured vegetables, plus supplements of beta-carotene, may also develop a yellow skin. However this should not be confused with jaundice, which obviously has an entirely different cause. One way to tell is that in jaundice the whites of the eyes also turn yellow, while in hypercarotenaemia only the skin turns yellow.

In jaundice, in addition to the coloration of the skin, there is another problem. Because the bile has not reached the duodenum, none of the usual bile pigments are released either. This means that fat digestion is adversely affected and that the stool, instead of being medium to dark brown, is a pale greyish colour.

The answer to this problem, yet again, is the Liver Detox Plan.

Liver Cancer

The liver is a common place to get cancer, both primary tumours,   meaning ones that started in the liver, and secondary tumours that   have metastasised from cancer in other parts of the body. Since the   liver deals with and stores so many toxins and since many of them   are carcinogens, it is hardly surprising that cancer of the liver is relatively common.

If you have liver cancer, the Liver Detox Plan should be considered as a part of your treatment, in combination with advice from your present practitioner.

Other liver diseases

There are, obviously, many other liver diseases, some common, some rare, but this is not the place to consider them all. However this section should have given you an overview of many of the things that can go wrong with your liver. Also, remember that many symptoms you have, though not perhaps obviously related to the liver, may in fact be so, and even extremely serious liver problems may be giving you relatively few warning signs. This is all the more reason why, if you have been living in a less than fully healthy way, you should follow the Liver Detox Plan.

Other Problems

An unhealthy liver can cause problems in a variety of other ways. Some of these have been alluded to elsewhere, others have not. It is also true that the various problems discussed below may not have originated with the liver, but that they are not being helped by the fact that your liver cannot do all that it should to help you deal with them. Keep in mind, though, that it is the contention of this book that there is almost no problem in your body that cannot be improved by improving your liver function, and that even if you have a problem that is not mentioned here, it could be beneficial for you to change your lifestyle and follow the Liver Detox Plan.

Allergies

Allergic reactions, or sensitivities, are on the increase. Thirty or more years ago relatively few people suffered from them, whereas today a high proportion of patients is found to be allergic or food sensitive to a variety of foods and substances or to have food or chemical intolerances. This may, in part, be due to our growing awareness of the problem and improved diagnostic techniques; but it may also be due to a true increase in incidence. I tend to favour the latter view. I know, for instance, that when I was at school none of my class suffered from asthma (commonly an allergic problem) and that, as far as I know, none of the girls in any of the other classes did either. Now it is common to find that up to perhaps a quarter or more of a class have breathing difficulties and asthma.

Allergic reactions and food sensitivities may be due to the additional chemicals and pollutants in the environment posing an increased challenge on the body, plus an accompanying decrease in the nutrient levels of many foods. There may also be other reasons, too, and a tired and unhealthy liver could be one of them.

Food allergies and sensitivities can start when foods are poorly digested, there is damage to the intestinal tract and the partially digested foods enter the bloodstream. They can result when there is a shortage of other nutrients, possibly due to poor intake but possibly also due to poor digestion and absorption of the needed nutrients. They can also occur when there are problems with the immune system, possibly also caused by inadequate nutrition.

We have already seen that your liver plays an important role in nutrition, the health of your digestive tract and your immune system. It also has to deal with any toxins produced during allergic reactions. For all these reasons the Liver Detox Plan can be of great help to you if you suffer from allergies, and this includes environmental as well as food allergies and food intolerances.

If you can improve your health by improving the health of your liver you may become less allergic and find that there are fewer foods and substances you have to avoid.

Anxiety Attacks

If your liver does not process lactic acid correctly, as mentioned earlier, this can lead to anxiety attacks, hot sweats, palpitations, stress, headaches and other symptoms of an anxiety or panic attack. This is one reason, if you do get anxious, to follow the Liver Detox Plan. It is also true that a healthy liver, with a full store of the B group vitamins, can help to calm your stress. A healthy liver can help you further by eliminating toxins and allergens that may be causing the problem. Many (hidden) food sensitivities create anxiety and tension, so can hormones that are not properly dealt with. An excess of thyroxine, for instance, can make you feel wound up, tense and anxious. Many toxins can also cause anxiety.

Brain Fog

Is your mind less clear than it used to be? Do you forget things, find that your concentration is slipping and get muddled more easily than you used to? It may not be your brain's fault that your mind is in a fog, it may be the result of a toxic system and a toxic liver. Once you have followed the Liver Detox Plan you will feel generally more alert, more 'clear' and more energetic and this includes your brain.

Cancer

The very word 'cancer' strikes fear in many hearts. No one wants to get cancer and few people expect it will happen to them, yet one in four people dies from cancer. Everyone is surrounded by chemicals and toxins that are carcinogenic and it has even been estimated that some individual cells in everyone succumb to carcinogens hundreds, even thousands, of times a day, but that a healthy immune system eliminates them, so you remain healthy. A healthy liver is a vital part of your protective system and so it can help to prevent the occurrence of this dreadful disease.

Candida

Candida albicans, a mould or yeast, occurs in everyone, but when it becomes a dominant species it can cause huge problems with multiple symptoms, both physical and emotional. The treatment is the subject of a book in itself (*Overcoming Candida* by Xandria Williams, Element Books), but you will help the situation a lot by improving the health of your liver. The flow of bile in the digestive tract and the proper peristaltic action will make the overall environment of the intestines an uncomfortable place for the candida to live.

If you do have this problem there will also be many different toxins generated, both in the digestive tract and within the rest of your body, that have to be dealt with by the liver. If they are not metabolised appropriately they can continue to circulate, causing you considerable harm and prolonging your symptoms. Many patients have found, however, that by following the Liver Detox Plan, within the constraints of a yeast-free diet, they have been able to reduce the severity of their symptoms and shorten the duration of their treatment.

Energy Problems

Your liver is involved in so many activities that affect your energy, both directly and indirectly, that it is difficult to list them all. It is vital for the absorption and transport of iron as well as its storage (the liver contains approximately 700 mg of iron) and iron, in turn, is essential for the transport of oxygen through the blood and its delivery to the cells that need it for energy. Your liver stores significant amounts of the B vitamins, also vital for energy.

Furthermore, as we have seen, your liver takes up spare glucose from the blood and builds it into glycogen which it stores. When the glucose is later needed for energy production it is then released back into the bloodstream. Your liver also helps to prevent hypoglycaemia and the energy slumps that accompany the associated drops in the blood sugar level.

The liver's role in maintaining normal levels of triglycerides and cholesterol in the blood can also benefit your heart and improve your circulation, further improving your energy. Its action in eliminating toxins from the body can enable you to mobilise stored fats more easily and thus lose weight more readily, and losing weight is commonly accompanied by an increase in energy.

If you are suffering from ME or Chronic Fatigue Syndrome (CFS), removing toxins from the body is a vital step. Once this has been done your energy level can improve significantly. It follows that if your liver is in poor health you are almost certain to feel tired and that if this situation is allowed to continue CFS could develop (see *Fatigue: The Secrets of Getting your Energy Back*, by Xandria Williams, also published by Vermilion).

Eyesight

If the liver does not perform properly, your chance of poor vision increases, as fructose, found in fruit and in table sugar (sucrose), can be converted into sorbitol and this can accumulate in the eye and lead to cloudy vision. A healthy liver can help, by increasing the conversion of fructose to glucose.

There is another way in which a faulty liver can cause eyesight problems. It is well known that you need vitamin A for your eyes, particularly to see at night, in the dark and to adapt from very bright lights, such as the headlights of an oncoming car, to the darkness that is left after the car has passed. Vitamin A is a fat-soluble vitamin and is stored in a healthy liver. To transport it through the blood a protein carrier molecule called retinol-binding protein is needed, as you may remember, and this is made in and mobilised from the liver; you will also recall that zinc is needed for the function of this protein. If your liver does not produce sufficient quantities of this protein and mobilise the vitamin A, not only will your eyesight be poor at night and in the dark, but it will also be poor in general and the surfaces of your eyeball and eye socket will become inflamed. You will also have other symptoms of vitamin A deficiency plus a possible build-up of vitamin A in the liver which can lead to vitamin A toxicity.

Headaches and Migraines

Headaches and migraines can both stem from an upset liver. Many are caused either by toxins or by allergens. If these are not eliminated by the liver in its detoxifying role then your headache can get worse as your liver function deteriorates. Migraines are commonly caused by allergens and we have already discussed your liver's role in relation to them.

There is another relationship between your liver and headaches and that relates to constipation. Many people find that their headaches are worse when they are constipated, probably as a result of the toxins entering the bloodstream. As we have already seen, a healthy liver and gall bladder can help to prevent constipation and thus help to reduce headaches.

Other headaches may be stress-related, and a healthy liver can help, in many ways, often indirectly, to increase your ability to handle stress without getting unwanted adverse symptoms. It can, for instance, do this by stabilising your blood sugar level and by removing lactic acid.

If you follow the Liver Detox Plan, get rid of the toxins, deal with the allergies, avoid constipation and improve your ability to handle stress, your headaches and migraines may become things of the past.

Heart Problems

An unhealthy liver can lead to increased blood lipoproteins, increased blood viscosity and circulation and heart problems, because as the amount of fat in your blood increases, your blood gets 'stickier' and so harder to push around the circulation system. This then puts an increased load on the heart.

Poor liver function can cause other problems by encouraging the formation of atheromas. An atheroma is the build-up of inappropriate tissues along the walls of arteries. Such formations are sometimes called deposits, though in fact they actually form within the artery walls. When they become calcified the situation is called atherosclerosis. There is debate as to the causes of atheromas but clearly the liver is involved in several ways. First, poor liver function can lead to increased circulation of cholesterol in the form of LDLs. The cholesterol *may* be doing the damage, though we do know that atheromas can form even when the blood cholesterol level is low. Equally, it is also possible that the culprits may be other components in the LDLs, such as the toxins they carry, toxins that could have been removed by a healthy liver. The atheromas can also be initiated by toxins that are not being carried by the LDLs, toxins that your liver should have extracted from your bloodstream and dealt with.

Remember, too, that the trans fatty acids found in hydrogenated fats and in margarine can block the production of the beneficial HDLs, lead to a build-up of LDLs and thus cause damage. Vitamin C improves this reaction.

If your blood cholesterol level is high, the way to get rid of it is to eliminate it in your stool. To do this you should include an increased amount of fibre in your diet.

By following the Liver Detox Plan you could be having a beneficial effect on your heart and circulation in several ways, and, since heart and circulatory disorders kill approximately 50 per cent of the population, this is extremely important and valuable accomplishment.

False Heart Attacks

Lactic acid build-up, as already mentioned, can lead to symptoms that mimic heart pain and problems, and even a heart attack. These symptoms can include sweating, left-sided chest pains and pain radiating down the left arm, high blood pressure and palpitations. So if you have been having these symptoms and continue to have these symptoms and your doctor tells you, after doing all the usual blood tests, that there is no evidence of a heart problem, it could be time to consider this possibility. And work on your liver as well as increasing your intake of B group vitamins and possibly supplementing with lipoic acid.

High Blood Pressure

As a student, the first time I heard the word 'idiopathic' was when we were taught about blood pressure problems. We were told that 1 per cent of the time high blood pressure was caused by kidney problems and 99 per cent of the time it was idiopathic. This latter seemed pretty important to me so I wanted to know what it was. Imagine my frustration when I learnt it meant 'occurring without known cause'. Fortunately, since then we have learnt more about the cause. We now know, for instance, that high blood pressure can be due to a deficiency of calcium or magnesium; it can also be aggravated by obesity.

You will also recall, from the section on hormones, that an excess of aldosterone in the blood, possibly caused by the liver's failure to remove the surplus, can cause high blood pressure by increasing the amount of sodium that is held in the blood and causing fluid retention.

Yet it is still true to say that much of the time the cause of high blood pressure is obscure or unknown. What we have found, however, is that when the diet is improved, in line with the Liver Detox Plan, and when this is accompanied by supplements to make good any remaining deficiencies, and when toxins are reduced, as in the Liver Detox Plan, patients have found that their blood pressure, if abnormally high, has gone down.

Obviously there are many possible reasons for this. One is the loss of weight that can occur when you reduce your load of toxins, another could be that the programme will in all probability increase your dietary intake of calcium, magnesium and potassium while decreasing your intake of sodium. Improving the health of your liver will also reduce the amount of fat in your blood, and this too could be an important factor.

So, if you have high blood pressure, do not be surprised if this falls when you follow this regime. If you are on medication you may want to have this checked as it may cease to be needed. Do make sure, though, that you follow the advice of whoever put you on the medication in the first place. Don't worry if your blood pressure is normal – following the plan will not cause this to fall to below normal levels. In fact if your blood pressure is low you may even find it rising back up to normal on this programme.

Fluid Retention

As you may remember, a lack of the proteins that live in the blood can lead to fluid retention. So if you suffer from this and all your doctor does is suggest that you reduce your intake of salt and take 'fluid pills', you might want to think instead about following this Liver Detox Plan to improve the function of your liver.

HRT, the Menopause and Related Problems

If you are lucky you can sail through the menopause with few, if any uncomfortable symptoms. Few women, however are this lucky, and most suffer from hot flushes, sweating, tension, irritability and many more symptoms.

For some women hormone replacement therapy is the answer to their prayers, at least in so far as it reduces the unpleasant symptoms. However for other women this treatment can also create new problems including mood swings, irritability and easy weight gain.

Many hormones, including the sex hormones, as we have seen, are based on cholesterol and that cholesterol cannot be broken down by the body. This means that every time you take in extra steroid hormones, such as HRT, you are increasing the work your liver has to do to get rid of them once their job has been done. In this regard, HRT is just another toxin or waste product for the liver to work on, at a time of life when it should no longer have to deal with all this oestrogen. Thus the Liver Detox Plan may improve the way your liver handles the HRT and decrease some of the unwanted side-effects it can cause.

On the other hand, HRT may reduce your liver's capacity to deal with other toxins, and result in symptoms that stem from them, so again, the Liver Detox Plan will produce benefits.

Some women refuse to take HRT even though they find the menopausal symptoms uncomfortable. The Liver Detox Plan can also help here, by helping to improve overall metabolism and hormone balance.

Hypoclycaemia

Hypoglycaemia (low blood sugar) has been mentioned several times already and it is time to provide a brief outline of what it is and what symptoms occur. As already explained, your blood sugar level should be kept within a narrow range. If it falls below this level hormones, such as adrenaline and others that are less well known, are activated. They travel through your bloodstream and trigger the release of glucose from tissues back into the blood. Some of this glucose comes from glycogen stored in the liver. If this fails, and your blood sugar level remains low, many extremely unpleasant symptoms will result. They include fatigue, a hollow/hungry feeling, including a craving for sugar, trembling, headaches, dizziness, mood swings, anxiety, irritability, depression and more, all contributing to a very uncomfortable experience.

Your sugar balancing mechanism can fail for a number of reasons, one of them being that your adrenal glands may be exhausted, in which case you need increased amounts of the B group vitamins, particularly pantothenic acid or vitamin B5, and vitamin C. Some of these, as we have seen, can come from the liver. Your adrenals may also be exhausted due to a heavy stress load, and this stress can be physical and chemical as well as emotional. Many circulating toxins can stress your adrenal glands – toxins that can be reduced by both decreasing their intake and by improving your liver's ability to get rid of them, both of which will happen on the Liver Detox Plan.

All this means that the sugar cravings, 'energy dumps' and erratic mood swings can be a thing of the past once your liver's function is improved and it can work to balance your blood sugar level.

The Immune System

Since your liver is an important part of your immune system, it follows that if it is compromised your immune system will be weakened and you will be increasingly prone to catching infections and getting sick. This means that after the three to six weeks on the Liver Detox Plan you may well find that you are getting fewer colds, avoiding the flu and escaping any other infections that are about.

Mood Swings

You're nicer than you think. It's true that much of what you say and do is dictated by your personality. However it is also true that many of your moods and emotions are affected by the chemistry going on in your brain. When that chemistry is faulty, your personality is affected.

There are many toxins that can adversely affect your health in this way. They include the results of a candida overgrowth and of allergic reactions or food sensitivities, both already discussed. They also include all the organic substances your liver has to deal with but may fail to process if it is unhealthy.

To take a specific example, if you think back to the way the liver is involved in getting rid of hormones once they have done their job you will recall that adrenaline and noradrenaline can, if your liver is not performing properly, be converted into compounds that can cause not only mood swings, but also psychiatric problems such as schizophrenia.

Detox your liver and you can be the person you really want to be – calmer, more relaxed and happier.

Osteoporosis

Osteoporosis is, essentially, the loss of calcium from your bones and a decrease of the amount of bone present. There may be pain in the bones, particularly in the spine, and there is an increased tendency for the bones to break. To maintain healthy bones calcium is needed, and vitamin D is needed for the absorption of calcium. Remember that vitamin D comes from two sources, either the diet or the action of the ultra-violet light in sunlight on the skin and the resulting conversion of a cholesterol derivative into the vitamin.

The liver plays a critical role in vitamin D metabolism. If your liver does not convert it successfully, then no matter how much calcium or vitamin D you swallow, you will not absorb it successfully. Thus if your liver is sluggish you could be at increased risk of calcium deficiency and osteoporosis. In some people the conversion process is so poor that a supplement is needed to prevent calcium deficiency.

Overweight?

Are You Really Overweight?

With the Western world's obsession with slimness, many people think they are overweight when in fact they are just right. So the first thing is to find out whether or not you really do need to lose weight. There are all sorts of ways of doing this:

- You can compare your weight and height with various tables issued, commonly, by insurance companies.
- You can focus on your body fat level, looking at skin-fold thickness. There are also special computerised weighing machines that will help you do this.
- However there is also a simple method you can use at home and for which you don't need any special equipment. All you have to do is work out the following calculation:
  1 Determine your height in metres and your weight in kilograms.
  2 Multiply your height by itself and divide the result into your weight and this will give you your body mass index or BMI.
  For females: A BMI less than 19 is underweight, 19–25 is normal, 25–29 is overweight and greater than 29 is obese
  For males: A BMI less than 20 is underweight, 20–26 is normal, 26–30 is overweight and greater than 30 is obese

Here are some examples:

Weight 60 kg, height 1.60 m, BMI: $= \dfrac{60}{1.6 \times 1.6} = 23.44$

You're fine as you are.

Weight 70 kg, height 1.60 m, BMI: $= \dfrac{70}{1.6 \times 1.6} = 27.34$

You are overweight and should lose some.

Weight 80 kg, height 1.60 m, BMI: $= \dfrac{80}{1.6 \times 1.6} = 31.25$

You're obese and must lose weight.

Weight 44 kg, height 1.60 m, BMI: $= \dfrac{45}{1.6 \times 1.6} = 16.28$

You are underweight and should gain weight.

So You Are Overweight

In our world of plentiful foods, luscious snacks and tempting cheats it was shown in one study that at any one time, 48 per cent of women were on a diet or 'watching their weight' and that 96 per cent of women go on a diet at some time in their life. It seems the figures for men are somewhat lower, perhaps because there are fewer social pressures on them to be slim.

Most diets fail, mainly because there is the underlying assumption that when you have finished the diet you can go back to your old ways. You can, but your weight will also go back to its old ways. Some people 'yo-yo' diet or follow a cycle made up of dieting, losing weight, going back to their old eating patterns, gaining their weight back and then starting all over again, others simply give up.

Some people come into my office and tell me that, no matter what they do, they can't lose weight. Some of these are cheating or fooling themselves and not actually reducing their caloric intake, but others do reduce their caloric intake drastically yet find the weight still does not come off.

There are at least two reasons for this low-calorie diet failure. One relates to your metabolic rate. When you eat fewer than about 800 calories per day your metabolism starts to slow down. This is a survival mechanism and was all very well in cavewoman days where lack of food intake could mean reduced ability to hunt and gather more food, leading eventually to death. Then, as a survival mechanism, the body became economical in the way it used what it had. Today this is a hindrance to survival, as increased body weight is associated with an increase in heart related disorders, diabetes, cancer and other degenerative diseases.

Toxins Are Stored in your Fat Deposits

The second reason these low-calorie diets don't always work is pertinent to our discussion of the liver and relates to toxins in the body. Most toxins taken in with food and drink or through the lungs are fat soluble. It would, after all, be stupid to use water-soluble pesticides on growing crops, they would be washed off in the next rain. Using water-soluble substances on fruit to increase their gloss would be a short-term project whereas waxes ensure that the fruit remains glossy to look at. These waxes may not be good for you, but they have visual appeal to the shopper, who continues to fall for the trick. Similarly most food additives and other toxins that we take in are fat soluble. All these fat-soluble toxins go to the liver. The liver does its best to deal with them, break them down, render them safe or expel them via the gall bladder. Some, after various changes, leave the body in the urine.

If your liver is overloaded, or if it is under-functioning, these toxins may be stored rather than processed. Because they are fat soluble, the obvious place to store them is in the fat stores of the body. This is the adipose tissue that makes up the extra padding and those rolls of fat you are trying to lose. In its wisdom, your body realises that if this toxin-laden adipose tissue is broken down, the toxins in it will be released and circulate throughout the body and brain, causing a variety of toxic symptoms. In self-defence, therefore, these tissues seem to become resistant to breakdown.

If you want to lose weight there are several reasons why the Liver Detox Plan will make that easy:

- You will be removing these toxins from your body and therefore from your adipose tissues.
- You will be cutting out all the high-calorie, high-fat and high-sugar foods.
- You will be increasing your fibre intake and the intake of bulky foods, so will feel full after eating fewer calories.
- You may reduce your sugar cravings, one of the urges that breaks many dieters' will-power.
- You will be increasing your level of carnitine, either by taking carnitine or methionine and lysine and/or by eating a diet rich in these nutrients. This in turn will improve the ability of your cells to take up and use fats from the bloodstream, converting them into energy. (You will recall that if carnitine is deficient the fats from your adipose tissue may be mobilised but unable to enter the cells, so they return to the adipase tissues and you feel hungry and tired and gain weight.)
- You will be taking supplements to ensure you have an adequate amount of all the nutrients you need.

This latter reason deserves some explanation. You only have one appetite switch in the brain and it can be either on or off. Logically, you might think that when you have eaten a sufficient quantity the switch goes off and you stop eating. However it is not so straightforward. If you are lacking in a number of nutrients, such as vitamins or minerals, the switch can stay on, even if you have eaten more than sufficient food to give you all the calories you need. You may well have had the experience of eating a large meal, knowing you are full, yet still feeling hungry for something, though you're not quite sure for what. That is your body telling you that the quality of the food was not up to standard and that certain nutrients were missing. When you make sure, by the quality of both your diet and the supplements you take, that you get all the nutrients you need, this type of false hunger can be a thing of the past.

Premature Ageing

No one wants to get old, and certainly not before their time. Yet if you let your liver become unhealthy you are likely to experience a lot of the degenerative diseases associated with age. These range from heart attacks and cancer to diabetes and arthritis and they include premature ageing of the skin and poor hair health.

As if that wasn't enough, unless encouraged by being given all the nutrients it needs and spared the toxins it does not need, your liver can actually decrease in size with age. This of course means it can do its job less well. So, if you want to look young and vibrant, with a clear skin and slim and supple body, it is important that you treat your liver well. Start this Liver Detox Plan at any age, but be particularly sure to follow it as you get older, unless you want to get older even faster.

Skin Problems

An unhealthy liver can lead to signs of premature ageing of the skin and it can also lead to acne, greasy skin, eczema, dermatitis and other skin problems. Acne can be worsened when you eat a poor diet and when you are constipated. Remember the vital role the liver has to play in helping to prevent constipation.

Acne can also result from the changes in hormonal levels that occur at puberty and the resultant increase of sebum produced by the cells that are near hair follicles, followed by bacterial infections and the production of the characteristic white or yellow pus. You need a healthy liver to metabolise these hormones and to prevent a build-up of any excess, otherwise the problem can be aggravated.

You may be thinking that surely teenagers don't have liver problems. Sadly they do. The modern diet of processed foods and fast takeaway meals, with an inadequate nutrient content, to say nothing of the toxins and other substances it contains that impact on the liver, are sufficient to cause problems with the liver at almost any age.

Eczema and dermatitis, meanwhile, are commonly the result of allergic reactions and we know that these can be reduced if your liver health is improved.

Tests for your Liver

How do you know what state your liver is in? The chemical blood tests done by your doctor, on one or more small vial of blood, will pick up serious structural problems. They are generally for liver enzymes and these only enter the blood in significant quantities when there is significant structural liver damage. Initial functional deficiencies will not lead to raised blood enzyme levels. By the time these enzyme levels are showing significant abnormalities, your liver is already seriously under stress. This means that a negative test from your doctor does not necessarily mean that you liver is in excellent shape.

It is therefore fortunate that there are several other simple tests that can be done to give you early warning signs if things are not quite as they should be, and that these will show results some considerable time before the medical tests show anything. These *are* early warning signs and it is important that you pay heed to them and do not wait for the medical blood tests to show results. Don't, as one patient said to me, say to yourself that the symptoms are minor, you can live with them, and so fail to take appropriate corrective action. By waiting until there is major damage accompanied by major symptoms you are creating serious problems for yourself. It is much easier to prevent problems than to solve them.

Checklist

The first thing you can do is look at the following checklist of the symptoms that could indicate that your liver is under-functioning. The more of these symptoms you have, the greater is the likelihood that your liver is under strain. Score the results and find out how important this detox programme is for you.

(Please note that there can also be other reasons for these symptoms. If the symptoms disappear once you are on the Liver Detox Plan you can probably relax, but if they don't you would be wise to look for and find the alternative cause and treat the problem accordingly.)

Ageing: premature
Allergic symptoms: new or increased allergic reactions
Brain: brain fag, poor memory and concentration, depression, mood swings, headaches, migraines
Cardiovascular system: high blood pressure, fluid retention, palpitations

Digestive system: coated tongue, bad breath, indigestion, bloating, nausea, intolerance of fat-rich foods, candidiasis, constipation, alternating constipation and diarrhoea, pale coloured stools, stools that float, stools that don't flush easily, fatty residue round the bowl, bloating and flatulence

Drugs: reduced tolerance to alcohol, unexpected hangovers, abnormal reactions to recreational drugs, increased side-effects from medical drugs

Emotions: mood swings, irritability, depression, anxiety, panic attacks

Endocrine: erratic blood sugar levels leading to hypoglycaemia and its associated symptoms including sugar cravings, mood swings and energy drops

General: easy weight gain, difficulty losing weight, fatigue, ME or CFS, unusual body heat or flushing

Liver and gallbladder: gallstones, inflamed gall bladder, pain over right upper abdomen

Musculo-skeletal system: rheumatism and arthritis (allergies)

Respiratory system: rhinitis, hayfever, asthma (allergies)

Skin: hives, acne, eczema, dermatitis (allergies), grey shadows under the eyes

Tests to Do at Home

There are some simple checks you can do to test out your liver and gall bladder.

Take a Look

You may be surprised to discover that there are some signs you can see on the outside, simply by looking, that will tell tales on your liver if it is not performing correctly. Have a look at the soft skin around the lower side of your eyes and on your arms and legs. There should be no yellowish fatty lumps. If there are, they are probably also occurring inside, in the parts of your body you cannot see, and they are a sign that your liver is not dealing with fats correctly. Not only that, but these fat deposits will interfere with the organs and tissues where they are deposited, the fat may be clogging your arteries, and you will soon find other symptoms developing as a result.

Look for jaundice, yellow coloration of the skin and the whites of the eyes – this latter, remember, is what distinguishes jaundice (yellow eyes) from an excess of carotene (in which case the whites of the eyes stay white).

Checking your Gall Bladder

For this test you will need the help of a friend. Lie flat on the floor, on a table or on some other firm surface. Find the lower edge of your right-hand rib cage. To do this, feel for the flat bone that lies down the centre of your chest. At the bottom you will feel a bony ridge on each side going down and out at an angle of approximately 45 degrees. This is the bottom of your rib cage. Now ask your friend to lie their right hand flat on your right abdomen, below and alongside your rib line and with the thumb touching this rib. Your fingers will be parallel to your rib bones. You are now ready to start the test.

First of all, let them know that you want them to press really hard on your abdomen. If they are gentle, the test will fail. Your are going to take a preparatory breath in, then breathe out as far as you possibly can. At the same time they are going to press down, up, and slightly to your right-hand side, as if they were trying to push their hand up and under your rib cage. You will then breathe in, and as you do so your lungs will expand. At the same time they are going to do all they can to keep their hand in the same place, to stop if from rising up with your abdomen. This will have the effect of squashing your liver, more particularly, of squashing your gall bladder between your liver and their hands.

Obviously this will lead to a feeling of pressure and constriction. That is normal. However you may also feel a sudden sharp pain. This is not normal. If it occurs, your gall bladder is probably tender. It could simply be inflamed or you could have gallstones or there could be some other problem. This may go away once you have followed the Liver Detox Plan. Alternatively you might want to seek professional guidance as to what could be wrong.

There is another way of checking on your gall bladder. The level of bilirubin and bile acids in the blood may rise when these substances are not being correctly passed from the liver to the gall bladder and excreted as part of bile. If so, you will probably also notice that your stools are paler in colour than normal, lacking the usual bilirubin, and your urine is darker, as the circulating bilirubin tries to leave your body via that route.

Reflexology and your Liver

In the Chinese system of healing there are thought to be many energy lines, or meridians, running through your body, from top to bottom. Each of them passes through specific organs or tissues on their way and each of them terminates in your feet (and hands). This means that the lines that pass through your liver all terminate on the sole of your right foot (since the liver is on the right side of your body).

You can do this test yourself, or you can ask a friend to do it for you. Find the liver position on your foot and press hard (consult a reflexology chart). If all you feel is the pressure you are applying, your liver is probably healthy. If, however, you find this is a particularly sensitive area of your foot, compared to other areas, then this suggests that your liver is under stress and needs attention.

Many years ago, in Australia, where reflexology is less common than it is in the United Kingdom, a chap had come to see me about a problem that involved his liver and digestive system. At the end of the consultation he said, 'Oh, by the way, I also have a sore foot. Is there anything you can do about it or do I need to see a chiropodist?' He indicated his right foot, and without giving it much thought I picked it up and asked, 'Where does it hurt? Here?' while automatically checking the liver. He was a bit surprised that I had gone straight to the tender spot and even more surprised when I told him not to worry, I thought it would improve over the next week or two. Sure enough, at his next visit he was able to tell me that not only had his digestion improved but the pain in his foot had also gone.

Tests with Professional Help

Blood Tests

If you go to your doctor with a suspected liver problem they will almost certainly take a blood sample. This will then be analysed for a number of components including liver enzymes and various proteins and your doctor will be able tell you if you have a liver problem. Keep in mind, though, that by the time these tests show positive the problem *is* serious and treatment is urgent, and that a clear result, particularly if you don't feel well, does not clear the liver of involvement. You may still benefit from the Liver Detox Plan.

Liver Enzymes

Liver enzymes have technical names that reflect the compounds with which they work, however they also have simplified names or initials, which makes it easier to remember them, such as alkaline phosphatase (ALK. PHOS.) and transaminases (SGOT, SGPT). These are found in the blood at increased concentration when there is liver damage and increased death of liver cells, since these cells then release their enzymes into circulation. If alcohol is the main punishment you are giving your liver, the level of a different enzyme, called gamma-GT, may be raised, while the other enzymes remain at normal levels.

Blood Proteins
As we have already seen, one of the jobs your liver does is to convert the protein and amino acids you have eaten into specific proteins needed by the human body. Many of these proteins are needed for tissue building, for building the muscles and so forth, but some of them are needed by the bloodstream where they act as carrier molecules, clotting agents, form part of your immune system and so on. They include prothrombin, globulins and albumin, and if the levels of these are incorrect this also indicates a problem with your liver.

Blood Fats
An early sign of liver problems may be the amount of fat in your bloodstream. Unless you have just eaten a fatty meal, your level of blood fats, the triglycerides and cholesterol, should be maintained within the normal range. Your fasting cholesterol level should be 4.0–5.5 mmol/litre and your triglyceride level should be less than 2.0 mmol/litre. If either of these tests show an increased result then your liver could be at fault.

Summary

Isn't your liver amazing? If you are in any doubt as to the range of its actions, just look back at the table of contents to remind yourself. It is also worth doing this whenever you feel like cheating on the Liver Detox Plan. For you will feel like cheating from time to time, everybody does, because the suggestions mean, for most people, a significant change from their normal habits. But think of it this way. The greater the difference between what you are presently doing and what is suggested in the plan, the greater is the possible damage that has been done to your liver and the greater is the importance of this regime for your health.

There is almost no health problem that will not benefit from this Liver Detox Plan. We have considered many of them here, but certainly not all. You may have a simple short-term health problem that can be dealt with by this programme. On the other hand you may have 'tried everything' and may have suffered for years from a variety of symptoms for which no one has found a specific cause and for which you have found no solution. You may be overweight, have allergies, hypoglycaemia, candidiasis or chronic fatigue that have not responded to their individual treatments. This programme may be just what you need.

Good health.

Index

Page numbers in bold indicate main references to a subject.